Neuroimmunology

CURRENT TOPICS IN NEUROBIOLOGY

Series Editor

Samuel H. Barondes
Professor of Psychiatry
School of Medicine
University of California, San Diego
La Jolla, California

Tissue Culture of the Nervous System
Edited by Gordon Sato

Neuronal Recognition
Edited by Samuel H. Barondes

Peptides in Neurobiology
Edited by Harold Gainer

Neuronal Development
Edited by Nicholas C. Spitzer

Neuroimmunology
Edited by Jeremy Brockes

A continuation Order Plan is available for this series. A continuation order will bring delivery of each new volume immediatedly upon publication. Volumes are billed only upon actual shipment. For further information please contact the publisher.

Neuroimmunology

Edited by
JEREMY BROCKES
California Institute of Technology
Pasadena, California

PLENUM PRESS • NEW YORK AND LONDON

Library of Congress Cataloging in Publication Data

Main entry under title:

Neuroimmunology.

    (Current topics in neurobiology)
    Bibliography: p.
    Includes index.
    1. Nervous system. 2. Immunology. I. Brockes, Jeremy, 1948 –
        II. Series. [DNLM: 1. Nervous system—Immunology. W1 CU82P
v. 5/WL 100 N4935]
QP356.N4825   612.8   82-3679
ISBN 0-306-40955-0   AACR2

© 1982 Plenum Press, New York
A Division of Plenum Publishing Corporation
233 Spring Street, New York, N.Y. 10013

Printed in the United States of America

Contributors

M. JOHN ANDERSON   Department of Embryology
Carnegie Institution of Washington
Baltimore, Maryland

COLIN J. BARNSTABLE   Department of Neurobiology
Harvard Medical School
Boston, Massachusetts

ELLEN K. BAYNE   Department of Embryology
Carnegie Institution of Washington
Baltimore, Maryland

HARVEY CANTOR   Department of Pathology
Harvard Medical School and Sidney Farber
    Cancer Institute
Boston, Massachusetts

LINDA L. Y. CHUN   Department of Pathology
Harvard Medical School and Sidney Farber
    Cancer Institute
Boston, Massachusetts

DOUGLAS M. FAMBROUGH   Department of Embryology
Carnegie Institution of Washington
Baltimore, Maryland

JOHN M. GARDNER   Department of Embryology
                         Carnegie Institution of Washington
                         Baltimore, Maryland

ZACH W. HALL   Division of Neurobiology
                         Department of Physiology
                         University of California
                         San Francisco, California

REGIS B. KELLY   Department of Biochemistry and
                             Biophysics
                         University of California
                         San Francisco, California

WILLIAM D. MATTHEW   Department of Physiology
                         University of California
                         San Francisco, California

RHONA MIRSKY   MRC Neuroimmunology Group
                         Department of Zoology
                         University College London
                         London, England

MICHAEL B. A. OLDSTONE   Department of Immunopathology
                         Scripps Clinic and Research Foundation
                         La Jolla, California

ERIC OUTWATER   Department of Physiology
                         University of California
                         San Francisco, California

LOUIS F. REICHARDT   Department of Physiology
                         University of California
                         San Francisco, California

RICHARD L. ROTUNDO   Department of Embryology
                      Carnegie Institution of Washington
                      Baltimore, Maryland

MELITTA SCHACHNER   Department of Neurobiology
                      University of Heidelberg
                      Heidelberg, Federal Republic of Germany

LARISA TSAVALER   Department of Physiology
                      University of California
                      San Francisco, California

ERIC WAKSHULL   Department of Embryology
                      Carnegie Institution of Washington
                      Baltimore, Maryland

Preface

Neuroimmunology could be defined as the application of immunological methods to problems in neurobiology but such a definition is so all-encompassing as to be unhelpful. It is not a precisely circumscribed discipline but it seems worthwhile at the outset to point to three of the major areas of activity.

One rather early use of the term was in connection with studies on the immune response to antigens in the nervous system. This includes topics such as autoimmunity in the central and peripheral nervous systems, the response to neural tumors or viral infections, and the immunopathology of such processes. Although not at the forefront of the currently fashionable preoccupation with neuroimmunology, this area continues to be a vital and interesting one from both clinical and basic perspectives.

A second very active area is the exploitation of antibodies to identified components of neural cells, and in particular to those molecules involved as neurotransmitters, in transmitter synthesis and breakdown, and as synaptic receptors. The immunohistochemical detection of these antigens has led to new insights into the functional organization of the nervous system, and reference to such studies is almost a *sine qua non* for discussions of most central and peripheral synapses.

The third area has its intellectual and practical antecedents in the discipline called cellular immunology—the study of different classes of lymphocyte and their functional interactions. As discussed in this volume by Chun and Cantor, the considerable advances in cellular immunology in the last fifteen years have in large part depended on the use of antisera to marker antigens, generally on the cell surface, which are confined to particular subpopulations of lymphocytes. A distinctive methodology has developed around the derivation and assay of such antisera, and their exploitation for identifying and purifying the different classes of T and B cells. The derivation of these reagents after immunizing with complex mixtures of antigens has been revolutionized by hybridoma technology. It is important to note that many of the marker antigens which have been so valuable in cellular immunology are molecules whose function is unknown, at least initially. The study of cellular heterogeneity among neurons and glia is, at one level or another, a basic preoccupation of neurobiologists. It is therefore a natural development to use the methodology of cellular immunology firstly to reinforce or refine traditional classifications based largely on anatomy or transmitter type, and secondly to seek new identities and differences between cells as an expression of fundamental aspects of development and organization.

This collection of essays reflects all of these interests. The authors' viewpoints are different, varying from studies on components of a particular synapse or cell surface, to an analysis of cell markers in the nervous system or particular areas of the brain, and to considerations of autoimmunity and the immune response that were referred to above. Together they provide a strong case for why neuroimmunology is currently so interesting and exciting, and also why it seems to be so promising for tackling some of the traditionally intractable problems in neuroscience.

I should like to thank all of the authors for their contributions, and Samuel H. Barondes for his excellent advice as series editor.

Jeremy P. Brockes
Pasadena, California

Contents

1

Immunology of the Neuromuscular Junction

REGIS B. KELLY and ZACH W. HALL

1. INTRODUCTION

Although the vertebrate neuromuscular junction has surely been the most intensively studied synapse in the nervous system, we know remarkably little about its structure and function at a molecular level. One simple reason for this is that the junction forms only a miniscule part of the total muscle tissue, and methods have not been devised for its purification as an intact structure. Isolation of any molecular component of the synapse is thus a formidable task. The only protein that has been extensively purified from the neuromuscular junction is the acetylcholine receptor (AChR); even in this case, the small amount of protein that can be obtained limits severely the kinds of experiments that can be done.

Because the neuromuscular junction is inaccessible to biochemical analysis, antibodies have become, and will continue to be, unusually important tools in its investigation. Components of the junction that cannot be detected or localized by direct assay can be identified and assayed by immunohistochemical methods. Two factors increase the power of this approach. The first one is the homology between the

REGIS B. KELLY · Department of Biochemistry and Biophysics, University of California, San Francisco, Calif. 94143. ZACH W. HALL · Division of Neurobiology, Department of Physiology, University of California, San Francisco, Calif. 94143.

vertebrate neuromuscular junction and the synapses in the electric organs of various fish. Because the electric organs receive dense innervation and are abundantly available, antibodies can be made to macromolecules purified from these tissues and then used to study the neuromuscular junction. This approach has been most thoroughly applied with respect to the AChR. The ready availability of purified receptor from *Torpedo* has made the production of antibodies to it a routine matter. These sera cross-react with the mammalian receptor; their use has been of enormous importance in advancing our understanding of the pathophysiology of the neuromuscular junction.

The second important factor is the recent development of the monoclonal technique. Antibodies can now be made to unidentified or partially purified components of the junction. Beyond simply identifying the macromolecules that are present, monoclonal antibodies (mAbs) provide extremely precise and well-defined reagents that can be used to intervene in functional or developmental processes or to define the role of particular parts of macromolecules. The potentiality of this approach is only beginning to be realized.

In this article, we describe the elements of the neuromuscular junction to which antibodies are currently available. We also emphasize the various uses to which these antibodies can be put. In some cases, they have been used to identify molecular components of the synapse for which no other assay exists, or to show that molecules found elsewhere in the body are also present at the synapse. They have been useful in structural studies of synaptic molecules, even sometimes as inhibitors of function. They have been used as markers of synaptic function and to purify synaptic components. They can be used as developmental markers. The conclusion we wish to draw is that many molecular aspects of the neuromuscular junction which were once considered unapproachable are now accessible by immunological methodology.

2. STRUCTURE OF THE NEUROMUSCULAR JUNCTION

The three parts of the neuromuscular junction (Fig. 1) to which we will pay attention are the nerve terminal, the synaptic cleft, and the postsynaptic membrane with its underlying structures. The presynaptic terminal is specialized for the synthesis, storage, and release of the transmitter ACh, and for the uptake of its precursor, choline. Morphologic specializations include synaptic vesicles and specialized sites around which vesicles are clustered on the membrane facing the muscle surface. These regions, called active zones (Couteaux and Pecot-De-

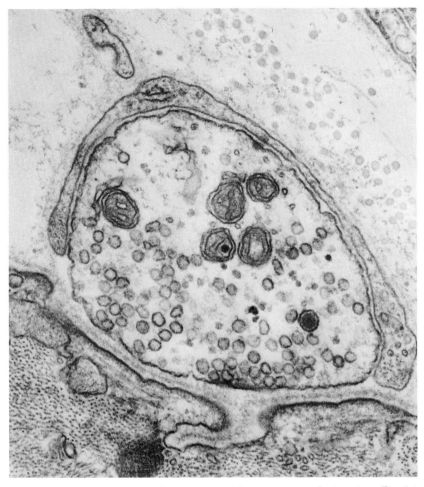

Figure 1. Electron micrograph of cross-sectional frog neuromuscular junction. (Reprinted from Sanes *et al.*, 1980.)

chavissine, 1970), are thought to be the sites of transmitter release (Heuser *et al.*, 1979) and are positioned exactly opposite the folds in the postsynaptic membrane. In thin section, they are characterized by a small amount of dense material on the inside of the membrane. Freeze-fracture experiments demonstrate the active zones to contain a double row of particles that extend across the terminal. The motor nerve terminal is known to have a high density of voltage-sensitive calcium channels, and it has been suggested that the particles may correspond to these molecules. The structure and properties of the nerve terminal have recently been reviewed (Heuser and Reese, 1979; Ceccarelli and Hurlbut, 1980; Kelly *et al.*, 1979).

The synaptic cleft of the neuromuscular junction is occupied by a basal lamina (BL) that ensheathes each muscle fiber and passes between nerve and muscle at the junction. Within the endplate, projections of the BL extend into the postsynaptic folds; at the edge of the junction, the muscle BL joins that of the overlying Schwann cell. Although virtually ignored for years, attention has recently been directed toward the BL of muscle fibers by the elegant experiments of McMahan and his collaborators (Marshall *et al.*, 1977; Sanes *et al.*, 1978; Burden *et al.*, 1979). They have shown that during regeneration of adult nerve and muscle, the BL at the old synaptic site can direct differentiation both of the presynaptic nerve terminal and of the postsynaptic muscle membrane.

Very little is known about the chemical structure of the muscle fiber BL, particularly at the synapse which represents such a small fraction of the muscle fiber surface. By analogy with other BLs it is assumed to consist of collagen, glycoproteins, and glycosaminoglycans. In contrast to pre- and postsynaptic structures from which components can often be identified and purified on the basis of enzymatic or binding activities, almost nothing is known about the macromolecular components of the synaptic BL. Thus immunological methods assume unusual importance in the identification and study of these molecules.

One component of the synaptic BL has been identified: AChE. The evidence that the AChE in the synaptic cleft is associated with the BL is based on the studies of McMahan *et al.* (1978) using damaged frog muscle in which the plasma membrane of the muscle cell has been removed by phagocytosis. After damage only the BL remains, yet AChE activity can still be detected at old endplates. Antisera have been prepared to purified AChE from several sources.

The only component of the postsynaptic membrane to be so far identified is the AChR which binds the ACh released from presynaptic terminals. This binding reaction causes the transient opening (ca. 1 ms) of a transmembrane channel that is selectively permeable to the cations, sodium, potassium, and calcium. In muscle, where the postsynaptic membrane is thrown into elaborate folds, the AChR occurs on the crests of the folds, at a density of about 2×10^4 toxin-binding sites per square micrometer (Fertuck and Salpeter, 1974). In the electric organ of *Torpedo* the receptors are packed at a similarly high density: the entire surface of the electroplax is continuously innervated and is covered with AChRs. These have been visualized as particles of about 8 nm diameter by negative staining, by freeze fracture, and by freeze fracture followed by deep etching (Heuser and Salpeter, 1979). After negative staining, the particles appear to be composed of five to six subunits, to have a central pit, and to extend about 5 nm into the extracellular space. X-ray studies confirm this picture and suggest that the protein extends through the membrane (reviewed in Karlin, 1980).

Underlying the postsynaptic membrane of muscle cells and *Torpedo* electrocytes is a dense filamentous network. At the frog neuromuscular junction, bundles of filaments, consisting mostly of intermediate filaments, but also containing microfilaments, underly the folds of the postsynaptic membrane and are aligned with them (Couteaux and Pecot-Dechavassine, 1968; Ellisman et al., 1976; Hirokawa and Heuser, 1980). Underneath the postsynaptic membranes of *Torpedo*, a loose, three-dimensional network is formed by filaments whose size is slightly less than that of the microfilaments of mammalian cells (Heuser and Salpeter, 1979). In addition to these filamentous structures, the underside of the postsynaptic membrane is seen to have a thick coating of protein which may correspond to the dense material on the inner surface of the postsynaptic membrane that is seen in thin-section microscopy. At mammalian endplates, this dense material occurs along the entire length of the folds and thus extends beyond the AChRs which are found only on the crests (Padykula and Gauthier, 1970). Most of the immunological studies on postsynaptic densities have utilized antisera to filamentous and other proteins, isolated from sources other than the synapse.

3. ANTIBODIES TO PRESYNAPTIC ELEMENTS

Aside from their obvious use in investigating specialized functions of the presynaptic terminal, antibodies to specific components of the terminals are also useful as markers. The developmental and trophic relations between nerves and muscles, for instance, are of intense current interest. Investigations of the ability of one cell type to induce or maintain specialized functions in the other requires reliable and convenient assays for that function. Antibodies are often suitable reagents for such purposes, one advantage being the ability to localize specific proteins to particular cells or parts of cells. Of the constituents known to be present in presynaptic nerve terminals, antibodies have been raised to three: choline acetyltransferase (CAT), synaptic vesicles, and the presynaptic plasma membrane.

3.1. Choline Acetyltransferase

The successful use of antibodies to dopamine β-hydroxylase (Helle *et al.*, 1979) and to glutamic decarboxylase (Saito *et al.*, 1974) to identify neurons in the CNS that contain norepinephrine and GABA, respectively, have prompted a number of laboratories to attempt to raise antibodies to CAT. Unfortunately, the task has proved unexpectedly difficult, and in spite of several early reports of success, it is only recently that the original aim appears to have been accomplished unequivocally. The problem has been a controversial one, almost willfully perverse in its difficulties. We detail some of these here because they illustrate par excellence the necessity for rigorous standards in the use of sera to localize proteins.

First, purification of the mammalian enzyme has been difficult to achieve. The most successful purifications have yielded preparations whose specific activities were in the range of 7–160 U/mg protein. With human brain as source, analysis of the purified protein on SDS gel electrophoresis showed a single band of 66,000 (Peng et al., 1980). Two purifications, both from bovine candate nucleus, gave two closely spaced bands of approximately 70,000 mol. wt. (Ryan and McClure, 1979; Cozzari and Hartman, 1980). In one case (Cozzari and Hartman, 1980) native gel electrophoresis also showed two bands, each of which contained CAT activity after elution, and it was assumed that these corresponded to the bands seen on SDS gels. A number of other preparations of the mammalian enzyme have been reported, but either have had much lower specific activities (Potter et al., 1968; Glover and Potter, 1971; Singh and McGeer, 1974; White and Wu, 1973; Shuster and O'Toole, 1974; Wenthold and Mahler, 1975; Chao and Wolfgram, 1973) or were grossly heterogenous (Rossier, 1976).

A second obstacle has been the difficulty of obtaining specific antisera to CAT. This is not a surprising problem when relatively crude preparations of enzyme are used as immunogen, but the production of specific sera to even highly purified preparations of enzyme have proved to be a challenge. Antisera produced in rabbits to the high specific activity enzyme (120–160 U/mg) described by Cozzari and Hartman (1980) and to the lower specific activity (7 U/mg) enzyme from human brain (Peng et al., 1980) gave a single precipitin line in a double diffusion test against purified CAT. Application by Cozzari and Hartman of a more stringent test of immunospecificity, namely immunodiffusion against contaminating fractions of protein that had been removed during purification, revealed small amounts of antibodies to other proteins in their sera. These results suggested that trace amounts of highly immunogenic components contaminated the purified preparation of enzyme. To remove the contaminants, antisera were made to the non-CAT-containing protein fractions, attached to Sepharose and used to adsorb the purified enzyme preparation. This step failed to alter the specific activity of the CAT preparation or its profile on native acrylamide gels, but successfully removed the contaminating immunogens, since antisera made to the resulting enzyme showed no reaction to components other than CAT. The antisera, which were made to each of the two forms of enzyme eluted from native gels, quantitatively precipitated CAT activity and gave a single precipitin line on double diffusion at all stages of purification. To establish that the precipitated protein was CAT, slices of the immunodiffusion gels were assayed and showed a peak of CAT activity that coincided with the precipitin line. Finally, Cozzari and Hartman showed that the amount of serum required to precipitate 50% of the CAT activity was the same at each step in the purification, demonstrating that the purified enzyme was immunologically identical to that present in the starting material. These experiments represent strong proof for immunospecificity.

The antisera to CAT produced by Cozzari and Hartman are the most thoroughly characterized of any yet described, but the only immunohistochemical localization yet reported by these authors is to neurons in the reticular formation of the pons and the medulla (Cozzari and Hartman, 1980). Interestingly, the distribution of stain within these cells is slightly different when seen by antisera to the two forms, suggesting that the forms can be antigenically distinguished. These sera have not been used with motoneurons; it will be interesting to compare staining of the cell bodies and terminals using antisera made to the two different forms of enzyme.

The antiserum recently raised to CAT from human brain (Peng *et al.*, 1980) is not characterized in as much detail as that of Cozzari and Hartman (1980) but does show a single precipitation line, containing enzyme activity, on immunodiffusion and immunoelectrophoresis. Using Fab fragments and the rabbit anti-CAT, (Peng *et al.*, 1981) specific staining is seen which has a distribution similar to that expected for cholinergic neurons. The antiserum stains the cell bodies of motoneurons in the rat spinal cord and of neurons in the neostriatum, accumbens nucleus of the diagonal band, medial septum, and olfactory tubercle. Stained motor terminals were also identified in the guinea pig diaphragm (Kimura *et al.*, 1980).

Evidence for the specificity of the antisera made to less highly purified preparations of the enzyme have been less good. For instance, antisera raised in guinea pigs to CAT purified from bovine brain have been shown both by immunofluorescence and by the PAP procedure to stain motoneurons (Eng *et al.*, 1974; Karen-Kan *et al.*, 1978). The immunogen was considered homogeneous because the serum gave a single band after immunodiffusion with a crude extract of caudate nu-

clei. Furthermore, the antiserum was shown to precipitate a single polypeptide chain of the correct size from the extract (Eng et al., 1974).
Unfortunately, the specific activity of the purified preparation, about
0.5 U/mg, was at best less than 1% of the most highly purified preparations described above (Chao and Wolfgram, 1973; Chao, 1975). This
means that the CAT either was almost completely denatured or was a
minor constituent in a highly purified preparation of another protein.
Rossier (1975, 1977) has suggested that the latter may be the case, pointing out that the calculated amount of CAT in caudate crude extracts is
not enough to account for the amount of protein precipitated by the
antibody. Also, although the antiserum does appear to be specific for
motoneurons in sections of spinal cord, it also stains cells in the cerebellum (Karen-Kan et al., 1978), where the amount of CAT is almost
undetectable (Goldberg and McCaman, 1967; Hebb and Silver, 1956).
This observation raises the unhappy possibility that the antiserum used
in these experiments was specific for a protein of unknown function
whose size is similar to that of CAT, and whose distribution shows
partial specificity for cholinergic neurons. The dilemma posed by these
experiments underlines the importance of rigorous and complete characterization of sera used for immunohistochemistry.

3.2. Synaptic Vesicles

The characteristic morphologic feature of the nerve terminal is the
synaptic vesicle. The synaptic vesicle membrane is thought to bud off
from the smooth reticular membranes of the axon, insert in the presynaptic plasma membrane during exocytosis, and be retrieved from it by
a coated-vesicle-mediated endocytotic step. The appearance of synaptic
vesicles in nerve terminals is a crucial step in synaptic differentiation.
If the synaptic vesicle contains unique antigens, then it should be possible to provide immunocytochemical evidence for the above scheme
and to use antibodies as markers of synaptic function and development.

The use of a purified organelle as an immunogen presents problems
that are in principal similar to those for a purified protein. The main
difference is the greater complexity of the organelle; it may contain
antigens that are unique and also those that are shared with other
organelles. Shared and unique antigenic determinants could reside in
glycolipids and proteoglycans in addition to polypeptide chains. To
generate a specific serum it is necessary to devise an adsorption procedure that removes antibodies to the shared determinants.

Antisera have been recently raised to cholinergic synaptic vesicles purified from the electric organ of *Narcine brasiliensis* (Carlson and Kelly, 1980). The purity of the vesicles was rigorously established by showing that the protein and lipid of the vesicles as well as the ACh and ATP contained within them showed a single peak when analyzed by velocity sedimentation, equilibrium density sedimentation, and electrophoresis (Carlson *et al.*, 1978). Analysis of the purified vesicles by SDS gel electrophoresis show them to contain eight major bands (Wagner and Kelly, 1979). Six of these copurify with the vesicles and may be specific to them.

The specificity of immune sera raised to the purified vesicles was tested in a solid-phase binding assay against purified synaptic vesicles and against a vesicle-free membrane fraction removed in the final step of vesicle purification. Some antibodies in the sera bound to both antigens showing that they recognized shared determinants. Adsorption of the sera with the vesicle-free membrane fraction removed antibodies to the shared determinants but left about half the antibody titer, presumably directed at unique determinants on the synaptic vesicles (Carlson and Kelly, 1980). The antibodies remaining after adsorption were demonstrated to be specific for the vesicles in several ways. When crude vesicle preparations were fractionated by glycerol or sucrose density gradients, a single peak of antibody binding was detected, that coincided with the vesicle peak. The ratio of ACh to amount of antigen was constant across the peak and was close to that obtained with purified vesicles. Finally, this ratio was shown to be constant at all stages of vesicle purification. These experiments suggest that synaptic vesicles contain antigenic sites that are not present to any large extent elsewhere in the electric organ.

Comparison of binding before and after sonication of the vesicles indicated that about half of the antibodies to synaptic vesicles were directed against antigens that were accessible from the cytoplasmic surface. After solubilization with a nonionic detergent, all the major vesicle components could be immunoprecipitated.

Immunofluorescence was used to see if antibodies to electric organ vesicles recognized related antigens in other species and in other tissues. Antibodies in the preadsorbed serum bound to motor nerve terminals in rat, chick, and frog muscle (Sanes *et al.*, 1979). The antigens recognized by the serum were probably associated with synaptic vesicles, since tissue sections were stained, but intact resting terminals were not (von Wedel *et al.*, 1981). In addition, the staining in terminals was intense, but was not detectable in cell bodies or motor axons (Hooper *et al.*, 1980).

Antibodies in the adsorbed serum bind not only to motor nerve terminals, but to a broad spectrum of terminals in the rat nervous system (Hooper *et al.*, 1980). These include cholinergic terminals in sympathetic ganglia, parasympathetic postganglionic nerves, hippocampus, and cerebellum and noncholinergic terminals in sympathetic postganglionic cells and in the posterior pituitary. Adrenal medullary cells are also stained. Other synapses in the cerebellum and hippocampus are not stained. What is shared by this diverse set of terminals and lacking in the unlabeled ones is unclear. The authors point out one feature common to terminals that contain the antigens: they store and secrete positively charged transmitters. Conversely, terminals lacking the antigens have neutral or negatively charged transmitters. Although it is not clear that the same antibodies are reacting in every case, these experiments demonstrate that the vesicles in marine rays and, by extension, the vertebrate neuromuscular junction share common antigens with vesicles derived from other cell types. They also illustrate that with the advent of appropriate antibodies it will be possible to divide nerve terminals into biochemically distinct subclasses.

Antibodies directed at unique membrane antigens are exceptionally useful for studying the biogenesis and fate of the membrane, even when the function of the antigen is not known. This is illustrated by their use in experiments on the mechanism of transmitter release from frog neuromuscular junction by von Wedel *et al.* (1981). Because the antisynaptic vesicle antibodies do not bind to intact nerve terminals, but do stain sectioned terminals, they reasoned that antigens associated with the synaptic vesicles are not normally present or accessible on the surface membrane of the presynaptic terminal. This allowed them to test a prediction of the hypothesis that ACh is released from stimulated motor nerve terminals by exocytosis, namely, that synaptic vesicle antigens will be transferred to the surface when vesicles fuse with the plasma membrane during transmitter secretion. This prediction was borne out. Stimulation of ACh release by lanthanum, which results in massive exocytosis, caused a dramatic increase in antibody binding to intact terminals. Control experiments established that lanthanum did not simply increase antibody penetration across the membrane. Unfortunately, increased binding could not be detected after electrical stimulation of the terminals, presumably because the prompt removal of vesicle membrane from the surface by endocytosis does not allow the antigens to accumulate in the plasma membrane. These antibodies should be useful in investigating vesicle membrane retrieval and processing in the terminal; by asking, for example, if coated vesicles contain synaptic vesicle antigens.

3.3. Other Presynaptic Antigens

Immunohistochemical localization of protein I, a protein associated with synaptic vesicles in the CNS, has been reported at the neuromuscular junction (Greengard and DeCamilli, 1981). Protein I was originally identified in synaptosomes from the mammalian CNS as a protein doublet whose phosphorylation was stimulated by cyclic AMP (cAMP). It has more recently been shown to also undergo calcium-stimulated phosphorylation mediated by calmodulin. Because intracellular concentrations of both cAMP and calcium are changed by nerve activity this protein has attracted attention as a possible mediator of activity-dependent changes in synaptic transmission. After immunoelectronmicroscopy using a second antibody conjugated to horseradish peroxidase, reaction product is associated with synaptic vesicles at a variety of synapses (De Camilli et al., 1979; Bloom et al., 1979). Thus, the antigen is widely distributed and may be present in all neurons. Immunofluorescence shows it to be present at the neuromuscular junction, where it is probably contained in nerve terminals (Greengard and De Camilli, 1981). Verification must await a more complete report, however.

Although the antibodies to synaptic vesicles described above do not bind to the plasma membrane of frog nerve terminals, they do bind to synaptosomes from marine rays. This forms the basis of their use in a bootstrap operation to produce sera that do react with frog nerve terminals. Synaptosomes from the marine ray Narcine were first coated with antisynaptic vesicle serum and then selectively adsorbed to polyacrylamide beads coated with goat anti-rabbit antibodies (Miljanich et al., 1982). Preimmune sera gave no adsorption. Hypotonic lysis and sonication of the bead-bound synaptosomes released the synaptosomal contents, leaving behind material rich in presynaptic plasma membrane and highly antigenic. An antiserum to this material bound an element of the frog neuromuscular junction, presumably the terminal, which disappeared on denervation (Fig. 2). Unlike the antiserum to synaptic vesicles, this serum binds to the outside of resting frog nerve terminals.

Antibodies to various constituents of the presynaptic nerve terminal membrane will be important tools in investigating the specialized activities of nerve terminals. The presynaptic membrane is an extremely active one, undergoing continual exo- and endocytosis. The orderly progression of these events must require considerable segregation of membrane proteins. Are calcium channel and choline transporter proteins, for instance, uniformly distributed on the membrane or localized to discrete regions? Do synaptic vesicle antigens have access to the entire

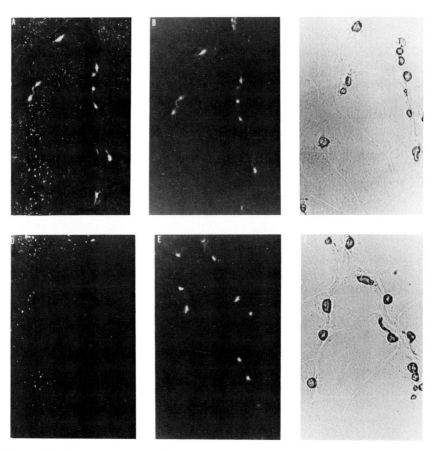

Figure 2. Antiserum to presynaptic plasma membrane from the *Narcine* electric organ binds to nerve terminals in cross-sections of frog cutaneous pectoris muscle. The binding of antibody is detected using fluorescein-conjugated goat anti-rabbit (A). Regions of antibody binding match regions of rhodamine α-bungarotoxin binding in the same section (B), and the regions of AChE staining in adjacent sections (C). Preimmune serum shows no binding (D) in sections where toxin binding (E) can be observed and where adjacent sections show esterase (F).

presynaptic membrane? If the synaptic vesicle membrane and plasma membrane are different, is there a separate vesicle carrying plasma membrane components to the nerve terminal? Antibodies to the two types of membrane will be of great value in sorting out questions on the synthesis and turnover of nerve terminals, as well as serving as markers for development.

4. ANTIBODIES TO COMPONENTS OF THE SYNAPTIC CLEFT

4.1. Acetylcholinesterase

The enzyme acetylcholinesterase (AChE) is highly concentrated in the synaptic cleft of the neuromuscular junction. Although the enzyme has not been purified from muscle, AChEs from the electric organs of eel and *Torpedo* have been extensively studied. Two general forms of enzyme are found in these tissues and in mammalian tissue as well (Bon *et al.*, 1979). The globular species consist of one, two, or four identical polypeptide chains, each with a single catalytic site. The tailed species are distinguished by a long (50 nm) asymmetric tail thought to contain collagenlike sequences. Attached to the tail are one, two, or three tetramers formed from the globular subunits (reviewed in Massoulie and Bon, 1982). Indirect evidence suggests that it is the tailed forms of the enzyme that are concentrated at the endplate. In some species, they are found only in regions of muscle containing endplates; also they appear at the same time as histochemical staining of endplates increases during synapse formation in adult and developing muscle (Hall, 1973; Vigny *et al.*, 1976; Weinberg *et al.*, 1981a,b).

Antisera to AChE have been made using both the mammalian enzyme and the enzymes from electric eel and *Torpedo* as immunogens. Since a simple and sensitive histochemical procedure is available for localizing the enzyme (Karnovsky and Roots, 1964), the pattern of staining observed with antibodies to the eel enzyme can be compared to the pattern of histochemical staining observed in eel electric organ, muscle tissue, and spinal cord and is found to be identical (Benda *et al.*, 1970; Tsuji *et al.*, 1972). Unfortunately, the strategy that has proved so useful in other cases, of using purified proteins from the electric fish to produce an antibody that can be used in mammalian tissue, has not been successful in the case of AChE. This was first found by Williams (1969), who made antibodies to the commercially available globular form of the eel enzyme; these failed to react with either erythrocyte AChE (Williams, 1969), or with muscle AChE (Z. W. Hall and M. Williams, unpublished experiments) by the criterion of immunodiffusion. Similar results were found by Gurari *et al.* (1974) and Greenberg *et al.* (1977), who tested antisera to the eel enzyme and to purified mammalian enzyme, using the more sensitive criterion of complement fixation, and found no cross reaction. In addition, Sanes and Hall (1979) failed to detect binding of antibodies to the eel enzyme at the mammalian neuromuscular junction.

Antibodies of AChE would be particularly useful if they recognized the tail portion of the molecule. They could be used to investigate whether the entire protein is assembled extracellularly and whether synthesis and secretion of the two portions of the molecule are independently regulated. Attempts to detect such antibodies in sera produced with tailed forms of the enzyme have so far proved unsuccessful. In each of the cases reported, preadsorption of the sera with globular forms of the enzyme completely removed reactivity with the tailed forms (Rieger *et al.*, 1973; Gurari *et al.*, 1974). This may not be surprising since the collagenous tail forms only about 5% of the total mass of the molecule and collagen is a notoriously poor antigen. Immunization with the isolated tail may be expected to be more successful; even this may be difficult, however, as large quantities of the purified tail portion of the molecule are not easily obtained. It may be possible to produce such antibodies using other immunogens. Anglister *et al.* (1979) have reported that guinea pigs immunized with rattail tendon collagen show a delayed skin reaction to tailed, but not to globular, forms of eel AChE. Likewise, when tested with radioiodinated forms of enzyme, antibodies from rabbits immunized with rat tail tendon collagen bound tailed but not globular species.

4.2. Basal Lamina

Because of the possible role of the BL in synaptic differentiation, there is great interest in identifying components other than AChE that might be selectively concentrated at the neuromuscular junction. It is not possible to approach this problem biochemically, because the synaptic BL has not been isolated from muscle. An alternate approach is to use antibodies. These not only allow identification of the macromolecules in the synaptic BL, but may provide tools to investigate its function. An account of monoclonal antibodies against basal lamina constituents of cultured muscle cells is given in Chapter 2.

Sanes and Hall (1979) immunized rabbits with immunogens derived from BL or related to it, and examined the resulting antisera for antibodies that bind selectively at the neuromuscular junction. Sera were tested by immunofluorescence on frozen sections of rat diaphragm using a fluorescein-labeled second antibody; endplates were identified in the same sections with rhodamine-labeled α-bungarotoxin. Three crude immunogens yielded sera containing synapse-specific antigens: anterior lens capsule, which had been solubilized in base; a basement membrane collagen fraction derived from anterior lens capsule; and a basement membrane collagen fraction from muscle. The two collagen fractions were produced by pepsin digestion and salt fractionation. In each case the synapse-specific antibodies were shown to be associated with the

BL, rather than the plasma membrane, presynaptic terminal, Schwann cell, or postsynaptic density.

After reaction with rat muscle sections, the antiserum obtained with solubilized lens capsule stained endplates, large blood vessels, and perineural sheaths. Endplate staining could be removed by adsorption with blood vessels, heart, or regions of muscle without endplates. In the latter case, the antibodies were presumably adsorbed by blood vessels in the muscle. These synapse-specific antibodies thus bind to other structures, but on the muscle fiber surface stain only at the endplate. In contrast to this serum, antisera to the two collagen preparations required preadsorption with endplate-free regions of muscle to reveal endplate-specific antibodies. In both of the latter cases, the synapse-specific antibodies stained only the neuromuscular junctions and could not be removed by adsorption with other tissues. Antibodies to the two collagen fractions could be distinguished from each other by a slight but consistent difference in the pattern of staining: the adsorbed antimuscle basement membrane collagen stained an area slightly larger than the endplate. Thus the synapse-specific antibodies in all three sera could be distinguished from each other. None of the three reacted with muscle AChE. The biochemical identity of the antigens recognized by these antibodies is not yet known. The antisera demonstrate that there are components of the BL that are uniquely concentrated or exposed at the synapse.

There also appear to be components of BL present only on the extrasynaptic muscle fiber surface. Using antibodies to purified proteins, J. R. Sanes (1982) has shown that collagen V and another collagenous protein occur in extrasynaptic BL, but are absent at the synapse. Collagen IV, laminin, and fibronectin are continuously distributed in synaptic and extrasynaptic regions (Fig. 3). Labat-Robert et al. (1980) have also used antibodies to purified proteins to show that fibronectin, laminin, and collagens IV and V bind preferentially to the innervated face of eel electroplax. No information is available about the distribution of these components at synaptic sites.

One application of the synapse-specific BL sera has been to study the appearance of the antigens recognized by these sera during synaptic differentiation. This is of particular interest, because experiments by Burden et al. (1979) have shown that the BL induces clustering of the AChRs at synaptic sites in regenerating muscle. Weinberg et al. (1981b) used the rabbit antisera to synapse-specific BL antigens decribed above to follow the differentiation of the BL during ectopic endplate formation in adult muscle. A foreign nerve, previously implanted in the soleus muscle, was induced to form new endplates by cutting the nerve to the

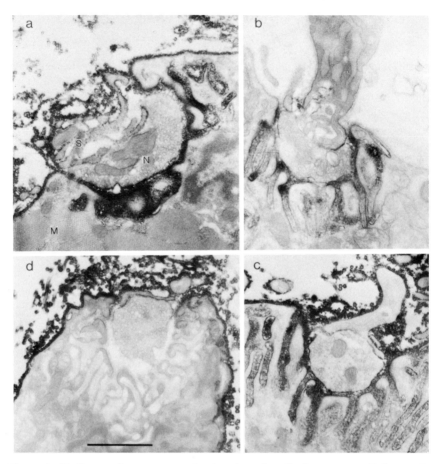

Figure 3. Binding to the neuromuscular junction of antibodies to extracellular matrix components. Antibodies to AChE (a) stain synaptic sites; antibodies to laminin (b) and fibronectin (c) stain both synaptic and extrasynaptic sites, while antibodies to proteins in a fraction from muscle connective tissue that is soluble in high salt (d) spare the synaptic sites but bind extrasynaptically. (Reprinted from Sanes, 1982.)

soleus. In this system, the first signs of functional transmission at the new synapses appear about two days after the nerve to the soleus is cut. The first appearance of synapse-specific BL antigens as detected by the antiserum to anterior lens capsule and the adsorbed antiserum to muscle basement membrane collagen occurred at about 6 days after nerve section. Binding was initially detected at only some endplates, but by 14 days all were stained. The time of appearance of the synaptic BL antigens coincided with that of endplate AChE, as judged by immunofluorescence, histochemistry, and the appearance of the tailed form of the enzyme in regions of the muscle where new endplates were being formed. The appearance of synapse-specific BL and AChE at the new synapses occurred distinctly later than the clustering of AChRs and the change in their metabolic turnover time induced by the foreign nerve. Both the density of receptors in the postsynaptic membrane and their turnover time had achieved adult values by the 6th day after nerve section. These experiments do not conclusively rule out a role for the BL in these processes since either different antigens or only small amounts of the ones detected could be required. They do show that the differentiation of the postsynaptic membrane and of the synaptic BL occur with different time courses, raising the possibility that the BL plays a more important role in regenerating old synapses than in forming new ones. It will be of interest to examine the formation of synapses in developing muscles with these sera.

5.   ANTIBODIES TO THE ACETYLCHOLINE RECEPTOR

The nicotinic AChR is not only the best characterized of the proteins at the neuromuscular junction, but one of the best characterized intrinsic membrane proteins found in eukaryotes. The wealth of information that we have about this protein is due both to the availability of a rich source—the electric organs of *Torpedo* and related fish—and to the discovery that certain snake neurotoxins bind the AChR specifically and with high affinity. These toxins can be radiolabeled to high specific activity and have been used to localize, quantitate, and purify the AChR both from electric organ and from muscle.

Purification of the *Torpedo* AChR after extraction from the membrane with detergent shows it to be a glycoprotein of about mol. wt. 250,000. It has a complex subunit structure with four different polypeptide chains, α, β, γ, and δ, with molecular weights of approximately 40K, 50K, 60K and 65K, respectively. These occur in the molar ratio of $2:1:1:1$. The α subunit appears to contain the ACh binding site as it is labeled by the affinity reagent MBTA. Two ACh binding sites and two toxin binding sites are found per 250,000 mol. wt. The AChRs of eel electric organ and of muscle appear to have analogous subunit structures to that of *Torpedo* AChR. Each has four different polypeptide chains with molecular weights that are roughly similar to those seen in *Torpedo*; in both cases the lowest-molecular-weight subunit is labeled by MBTA. In muscle a second subunit, shown by peptide mapping to a similar to the first, is also labeled by MBTA. In membranes from *Torpedo*, but not

Electrophorus or muscle, the AChR exists in the membranes as a dimer linked by disulfide bonds between subunits. Further details of AChR structure and regulation are given in two recent reviews (Fambrough, 1979; Karlin, 1980).

The AChR is also one of the membrane proteins whose immunology has been most thoroughly explored. Because the AChR can be easily purified and is highly immunogenic, a variety of antibody preparations have been available for its study. Although the snake toxins have provided some of the answers that in other systems have required immunological methods, antibodies have been extremely useful in studying aspects of AChR structure, localization, and metabolism. Studies of the immunology of the AChR have been given special impetus by the discovery that the disease myasthenia gravis is an autoimmune disease in which circulating antibodies to the AChR are thought to play a major role (for recent reviews, see Lindstrom and Dau, 1979; and Drachman, 1981).

5.1. Sources of Antibodies

In comparing different studies of the immunology of the AChR, it is important to bear in mind that at present there are three sources of antibodies to the AChR: those obtained by immunizing animals with purified AChR; those found in the sera of patients with myasthenia gravis; and the monoclonal antibodies made by hybridomas from immunized animals. We shall find that different determinants may predominate in the immune response according to the source. The choice of which antibody to use is therefore an important one.

5.1.1. *Animal Sera.* Antibodies to the AChR have been raised in goats, monkeys, rabbits, guinea pigs, rats, and mice by immunizing them with solubilized AChR purified from *Torpedo* or *Electrophorus* electric organ or from mammalian muscle or a muscle cell line. In each case, as originally observed by Patrick and Lindstrom (1973), animals develop a muscular weakness similar to that seen in myasthenia gravis in that it is associated with a decrementing EMG, and is relieved by cholinesterase inhibitors. This suggests that the animals produce antibodies to their own receptors, and analysis of the serum of the immunized animals shows this to be the case. In the case of immunization with xenogeneic AChR, the observed cross-reaction of the sera could be due to antibodies that recognize both the immunizing foreign receptor and the self receptor; alternatively, each receptor type might be recognized by separate populations of antibodies. In the latter case, since normal sera do not possess anti-AChR activity, it would be necessary to pos-

tulate that immunization with the foreign AChR stimulated production of antibodies specific for endogenous AChR.

Berman and Patrick (1980) examined this question in mice immunized with purified AChR from *Torpedo* by testing the ability of unlabeled *Torpedo* AChR–α-BuTx complexes to remove activity against mouse AChR–$[^{125}I]$-α-BuTx from mouse sera. In 60% of the cases, all of the antimouse AChR activity was removed; in the remaining 40%, however, antibodies appeared to be present that recognized mouse, but not *Torpedo*, AChR. In most cases, antibodies specific for the mouse AChR accounted for less than 10% of the total number of cross-reacting antibodies. Thus although some of the cross-reaction can represent the presence of a second population of antibodies, it is mostly due to individual antibodies that recognize two species of AChR. This was seen by Lindstrom *et al.* (1978*a*), who purified antibodies raised to *Electrophorus* AChR on an affinity column made with *Torpedo* AChR, and found that the purified antibodies had the same titer against both receptors. The purified antibodies retained some but not all of their cross-reactivity to muscle AChR, showing that there are several cross-reacting determinants.

These same authors have made what is probably the most complete comparison of the cross-reactivity of sera to the AChR. They examined the reactivity of AChR from different species with sera from a variety of animals immunized to AChRs from different sources. Although the sample size for each case is small, the general conclusion is that the sera are widely cross-reactive, with the highest titer always exhibited against the immunizing species. Serum from rats immunized against syngeneic AChR showed the most extensive cross-reaction. In general, mammalian AChRs appeared to share more determinants with each other than with the fish receptors.

The cross-reactivity of the antisera generated in an immunized animal appears to be under genetic control. Berman and Patrick (1980) made a systematic examination of the variation in cross-reactivity between mouse and Torpedo AChR among sera from different mouse strains immunized with *Torpedo* AChR. Despite variation between individuals within a strain, some strains consistently showed lower levels of cross-reactivity than others. Ten of 12 A/J mice, for instance, showed no detectable reaction with mouse AChR, while 9 of 9 AKR/Cu mice had titers at least 10-fold higher than background. The cross-reactivity was not linked to the ability to make antibodies since titers to *Torpedo* AChR were, if anything, higher in the A/J strain.

The extent of cross-reaction can also depend on the immunization schedule. In particular, after immunization with AChRs from *Torpedo* or eel, antibodies to mammalian receptor may appear later in the immune response than those to the immunogen and may require repeated inoculations to be detectable (Lindstrom et al., 1976a; Zurn and Fulpius, 1976; Lindstrom et al., 1979a,b).

The cross-reaction experiments emphasize the heterogeneity of the antibody response to immunization with purified native AChR. The antigenic complexity of the AChR is also seen in experiments with modified forms of the AChR. Antisera to native Torpedo AChR, for instance, contain antibodies that bind to the native protein but do not bind to AChR that has been denatured by treatment with guanidinium chloride followed by reduction and alkylation (Bartfeld and Fuchs, 1979) or by treatment with SDS (Claudio and Raftery, 1977; Lindstrom et al., 1978b). The latter case is particularly dramatic as fewer than 1% of the antibodies formed against native AChR are adsorbed by the denatured molecule. Thus, many of the antigenic sites on the receptor are conformationally dependent. Some antisera made against denatured receptor are composed almost entirely of antibodies that recognize the native protein as well (Bartfeld and Fuchs, 1977; Lindstrom et al., 1978b), while others appear to contain antibodies specific for the denatured receptor (Karlin et al., 1978). The heterogeneity of anti-AChR sera is also shown by trypsin treatment which removes some, but not all, of the determinants recognized by antibodies to the native AChR (Bartfeld and Fuchs, 1979).

Antibodies have been made in rats and in rabbits to the subunits of Torpedo AchR after their separation of SDS gel electrophoresis. Antisera made to each of the chains react with native AchR as well as to the subunit used as immunogen (Claudio and Raftery, 1977; Lindstrom et al., 1978b, 1979b). Indeed, in one case the concentration of antibodies titered against the homologous chain and against the native AchR by Lindstrom et al. (1979b) were almost identical.

5.1.2. *Myasthenic Sera.* The observation that AChR immunization produces a neuromuscular paralysis that resembles in many aspects the human disease myasthenia gravis has prompted investigation of the sera of myasthenic patients. Antibodies to human muscle receptor are found in 70–87% of cases. These sera, like those of animals immunized with AChR, show a wide spectrum of cross-reactivities (Lindstrom et al., 1978a; Appel et al., 1975; Aharonov et al., 1975). When tested against solublized receptors from various species, cross-reactivity of myasthenic sera with human and monkey AChR was highest, whereas that against electric organ AChR was poor (Lindstrom et al., 1978a). Cross-reactivity can also be demonstrated indirectly by the ability of myasthenic sera to cause symptoms of myasthenia in mice by passive transfer (Toyka et al., 1977) or to modulate the metabolic degradation of AChRs of mouse or rat muscle in culture (Kao and Drachman, 1977; Stanley and Drachman, 1978; Appel *et al.*, 1977).

It should be noted that serum from animals immunized with AChR is sometimes referred to as myasthenic serum if the animals develop symptoms of experimental autoimmune myasthenia gravis (EAMG). In this chapter, the term *myasthenic serum* refers only to serum from humans that have the disease myasthenia gravis.

5.1.3. Monoclonal Antibodies. MAbs to the AChR have now been made by several laboratories. These have been produced by fusion of mouse myeloma cells with spleen cells from rats or mice that had been immunized with purified *Torpedo* AChR (Gomez *et al.*, 1979; Moshly-Rosen *et al.*, 1979; Lennon and Lambert, 1980; Tzartos and Lindstrom, 1980; James *et al.*, 1980). In addition, preliminary reports of mAbs made to purified muscle AChR have appeared (Miller and Hall, 1979; Tzartos and Lindstrom, 1981). As would be predicted from studies on immune sera from animals, several of the mAbs to *Torpedo* receptor also recognize vertebrate muscle AChR. This has been seen both by binding of the antibody to solubilized AChR (Lemmon and Lambert, 1980; Tzartos and Lindstrom, 1980) and by the ability of antibody to cause myasthenic symptoms after passive transfer into recipient animals (Lennon and Lambert 1980; Tzartos and Lindstrom, 1980). One surprising feature of these experiments is that the proportion of mAbs to *Torpedo* AChR that also react with muscle AChR is much higher than might have been expected from the results on animal sera. Thus, Lennon and Lambert (1980) report that in different individual fusions 26–100% of the hybridomas made antibodies that recognized determinants common to both mammalian muscle and *Torpedo* AChRs; also, 9 of the 17 mAbs described by Tzartos and Lindstrom (1980) showed cross-reaction to muscle AChR from one or more mammalian or avian species. One possible explanation for these results is that the production of cross-reacting antibodies is normally heavily suppressed, but that in the protocols used for making mAbs the spleen cells are taken (3–5 days after the last injection of AChR in the two reports discussed here) before the mechanisms of suppression exert their maximal effect. If this is true, estimates of the relatedness of two AChR species by the degree of cross-reactivity measured with sera are apt to be in error. Curiously, in one study (Tzartos and Lindstrom, 1980) the affinity of the mAbs to muscle AChR appeared to be much lower than that for *Torpedo* AChR, while in the other (Lennon and Lambert, 1980) the affinities appeared to be in the same range (i.e., within an order of magnitude). As would be predicted from studies on whole sera, many of the mAbs (5 of 17) produced by immunization against native *Torpedo* AChR did not react with the denatured AChR, whereas all that were positive for denatured AChR also recognized the native form (Tzartos and Lindstrom, 1980).

The reaction of mAbs with individual subunits labeled with ^{125}I was tested by Tzartos and Lindstrom (1980). About half were found to react to the separated subunits. The subunit specificity of the remaining ones was tested by their ability to inhibit binding of the subunit-specific mAbs to the native AChR. Competition experiments revealed that a very large proportion of the mAbs were directed at a single site on the α-subunit. Gullick *et al.* (1981) have attempted to characterize further the binding sites for particular mAbs by investigating their ability to bind to defined proteolytic fragments.

5.2. Experimental Uses of AChR Antibodies

5.2.1. Subunit Structure of AChR. The problem of establishing the polypeptide chain composition of the AChR has been a particularly vexing one. It is only recently that investigators in the field are generally agreed that AChRs from *Torpedo* and *Electrophorus* electric organs and from mammalian muscle have homologous structures consisting of four different polypeptide chains. Perhaps because it is a membrane protein, the receptor is able to undergo considerable proteolysis without losing its native structure or ability to bind [^{125}I]α-BuTx (Klymkowsky *et al.*, 1980; Lindstrom *et al.*, 1980b). Thus there have been conflicting reports and much controversy over the number of chains in AChRs from different species.

Antibodies to the AChR have played an important role in resolving these issues. Initially, antisera were used to distinguish the four chains, providing important evidence that they were distinct and not derived from each other; further examination, using the more refined analysis that is possible with monoclonal antibodies, has revealed homologies between different chains.

Immunodiffusion and immunoprecipitation experiments with isolated ^{125}I-labeled chains showed that sera to individual chains are highly specific, although immunoprecipitation, the more sensitive method, also showed several cases of weak cross-reaction (<10%). The cross-reaction could have been due to cross-contamination in the immunogens or in the radioactive subunits with which the antisera were tested (Lindstrom *et al.*, 1979b). The chief conclusion from these studies, then, is that the four chains are immunologically distinct, consistent with the observation that all four have different peptide maps (Froehner and Rafto, 1979; Nathanson and Hall, 1979; Lindstrom *et al.*, 1979a).

The availability of mAbs allowed a more unambiguous test of the origin of the small amount of cross-reactivity that was seen with the sera to individual subunits. Tzartos and Lindstrom (1980) characterized the mAbs made both to native *Torpedo* AChR and to its subunits by their reaction with ^{125}I-labeled subunits. Although most were specific for a single subunit, two were found that bound two different subunits. One antibody prepared against δ also bound γ and a second, prepared against β, also reacted with α. In both cases, reaction with the heterologous subunit was weaker. The interpretation of these results obviously depends critically on the monospecificity of the antibody preparation. Tzartos and Lindstrom report that 10 different subclones of each hybridoma had the same specificity and that isoelectric focusing showed a single species of antibody. The cross-reaction therefore must arise from regions of homology on γ and δ and on α and β subunits. Because there is extensive homology in the sequence of the first 50 amino acids of each subunit (Raftery *et al.*, 1980), the continued production of mAbs to the AChR will probably lead to the discovery of other immunological homologies between the various chains.

The stoichiometry of binding of mAbs to the native AChR can give information about the stoichiometry of subunits within the receptor. In an initial study, Conti-Tronconi *et al.* (1981) examined the interaction between *Torpedo* AChR monomers (α$_2$βγδ), and several mAbs, using sucrose gradient centrifugation to characterize the products. One group of mAbs to the α subunits formed only 1:1 complexes with the AChR at all concentrations of antibody and receptor tested. In these complexes, the antibody was presumed to form an internal cross-link between the two α subunits in each AChR monomer. A similar stoichiometry was shown by a mAb that reacted with both γ and δ subunits. In contrast, other mAbs to the α subunit formed complexes of varying stoichiometries with the AChR. A plausible explanation is that the steric locations of the sites on the two α chains do not permit internal cross-linking, but allow intermolecular aggregates to form, as with complex antisera. A bivalent antibody that recognized only a single determinant on each AChR, as for instance on each β, γ, or δ chain, would be expected to form complexes in which the AChR/antibody ratio was either 1 or 2; no monoclonal antibodies of such specificity have so far been studied.

Antisera and mAbs to the isolated chains of *Torpedo* AChR have been used to test other AChRs for the presence of homologous subunits. Immunodiffusion experiments, for instance, have shown that sera to each of the four subunits of *Torpedo californica* recognize only the corresponding subunit in AChRs purified from several other species of marine ray (Claudio and Raftery, 1977). Eel AChR also has four subunits, each of which can be shown to correspond to one of the subunits in

Torpedo AChR. The subunits corresponding to α, β, and δ each react only with the appropriate corresponding antiserum. The fourth subunit is recognized both by antisera to γ and to δ and by a monoclonal antibody to *Torpedo* δ that cross-reacts with γ. As this is exactly the pattern of reactivity shown by the γ subunit of Torpedo AChR, this subunit presumably corresponds to γ (Lindstrom *et al.*, 1979b, 1980a).

Antibodies to all four *Torpedo* subunits have also been shown to react with AChR from mammalian muscle. Rats immunized with each of the isolated polypeptide chains from *Torpedo* AChR develop symptoms of myasthenia, have circulating antibodies to rat AChR, and show reduced levels of muscle AChR (Lindstrom *et al.*, 1978b). These results suggest that the muscle AChR has exposed on the cell surface components that share determinants with each of the four subunits. The observation by Berman and Patrick (1980), however, that xenogeneic receptor can cause the production of antibodies specific for the host receptor clouds the interpretation of these experiments. More direct evidence for recognition was shown by the ability of antisera to all four chains to bind to AChR from human or fetal calf muscle labeled with [^{125}-I]α-BuTx from human or fetal calf muscle. In each case binding was blocked only by the homologous subunit of *Torpedo* AChR (Lindstrom *et al.*, 1978b, 1979b). Although purified AChR from mammalian muscle has been reported to have four different subunits roughly corresponding in size to those seen in *Torpedo* (Boulter and Patrick, 1977; Froehner *et al.*, 1977; and Nathanson and Hall, 1979; but see Merlie *et al.*, 1977, and Shorr *et al.*, 1978), there is no direct proof that antibodies to each of the *Torpedo* subunits recognize determinants on homologous subunits of the muscle AChRs. The indirect evidence is quite strong, however.

5.2.2. Ultrastructural Localization of AChR Sites. Antibodies have been useful in identifying the AChR in the light and electron microscopes and in studying its disposition in the membrane. For purposes of localizing the AChR on cells and in tissues, methods employing antibodies to the AChR offer a supplement to the use of α-BuTx and antitoxin antibodies. Localization of the AChR to the endplates of adult muscle and to synapses in electric organ has been accomplished by identifying in the light microscope fluorescent, radioactive, or peroxidase derivatives of α-BuTx or by immunoperoxidase-staining unmodified α-BuTx bound to the AChR (Hartzell and Fambrough, 1972; Bourgeois *et al.*, 1972; Anderson and Cohen, 1974; Porter and Barnard, 1975; Daniels and Vogel, 1975; Lentz *et al.*, 1977). Autoradiography and immunoperoxidase staining of α-Butx in the electron microscope show that the AChRs occur largely on the crests of the elaborately folded postsynaptic muscle membrane (Fertuck and Salpeter, 1974; Daniels and

Vogel, 1975; Lentz *et al.*, 1977; Engel *et al.*, 1977b). Staining with exogenous antibodies to the AChR has not been reported at mammalian
muscle endplates, but Karlin *et al.* (1978) used antisera to eel and *Torpedo*
AChRs to stain the endplates in eel electroplaques by the immunoperoxidase method. The distribution of stain seen with both the light and
electron microscopes was identical to that observed by Bourgeois *et al.*
(1971, 1972) using immunofluorescence and high-resolution autoradiography. Direct and indirect labeling with ferritin were also attempted,
but apparently the ferritin conjugates failed to penetrate the synaptic
cleft.

Immune complexes at the endplates of patients with myasthenia
gravis have been detected by treating biopsies of intercostal muscles
with staphylococcal protein A that had been coupled to peroxidase. IgG
was detected on the postsynaptic membrane of muscles from myasthenic, but not from normal, subjects. The bound IgG had a patchy
distribution on the membrane, was associated with debris in the synaptic
cleft, and was accompanied by degeneration and simplification of the
postsynaptic folds. The complement component, C3, was detected on
the postsynaptic membrane of myasthenic, but not of normal, muscles,
by an anti-human C3 antibody coupled to peroxidase (Engel *et al.*, 1977a).

Antibodies have been used in several ways to identify AChRs in
membrane fragments from *Torpedo*. Klymkowsky and Stroud (1979) used
AChR antibodies immobilized on electron-opaque gold microspheres to
establish that the structures seen in the electron microscope to extend
out from the surface of *Torpedo* vesicles after negative staining corresponded to AChRs. In this case, the antibody provided a useful alternative to α-BuTx, which forms an unstable complex with gold beads.
Experiments in which antibody binding was visualized by direct and
indirect ferritin labeling also showed the extension of the AChR beyond
the membrane (Karlin *et al.*, 1978). When the primary antibodies were
labeled, ferritin was seen about 10–13 nm beyond the membrane, a
distance somewhat greater than the 8 nm found with antibodies to other
membrane proteins (Sternberger, 1974); when the secondary antibodies
were labeled, an even greater distance (15–20 nm) separated ferritin
from the membrane. In fact, the antibodies could be visualized directly.
Staining with unlabeled immune sera produced an electron-dense layer,
15–20 nm thick, on the outer surface of the membrane that was not seen
with normal sera. This is consistent with the suggestion by Rash *et al.*
(1976) that the fuzzy coat seen on the crests of the folds of myasthenic
muscle corresponds to bound IgG.

Antibodies have the greatest potential use in identifying parts of
the AChR other than the toxin-binding site. One example of this is the

use of antibodies to establish that the AChR traverses the membrane. Although Karlin *et al.* (1978) reported that they were able to detect antibody binding only to the external surface of *Torpedo* vesicles, Tarrab-Hazdai *et al.* (1978), using a ferritin-labeled second antibody, observed that open-membrane profiles often were labeled on both sides. They interpreted this to mean that the AChR extends through the membrane, exposing antigenic sites on both sides. This experimental observation was further refined by Strader *et al.* (1979), who devised methods for systematically exposing each side of an AChR-rich vesicle preparation. To expose the outside surface, vesicles were attached to cover slips pretreated with Alcian Blue. Sonication of the bound vesicles left only membrane that was directly attached to the coverslips and exposed the cytoplasmic face. The unsonicated and sonicated preparations were labeled with α-BuTx, followed by anti-α-BuTx, followed by protein A conjugated to hemocyanin. The large size of the hemocyanin allowed direct visualization in the electron microscope. Antibody to both α-BuTx and AChR bound intact vesicles; only anti-AChR bound to the exposed cytoplasmic face. In the latter case only one of six antisera was active, suggesting that the difference in results obtained by Karlin *et al.* (1978) and Tarrab-Hazdai *et al.* (1978) may have been due to differences in the specificity of the antisera used. Strader *et al.* (1979) were unable to detect any reaction of the positive serum with solubilized membranes that had been depleted of AChR, thus ruling out the possibility that antibodies to contaminating proteins bound to the cytoplasmic face of the membrane. They concluded that the AChR extends through the membrane, with the toxin-binding site on the outside.

These results have been confirmed and extended in a more recent study by Froehner (1981), who used a quantitative assay to characterize the location of sites recognized by several sera to *Torpedo* AChR. In two sera, raised against purified native AChR, 70–80% of the antibodies were bound by impermeable, right-side-out membrane vesicles containing the receptor. Thus, these sera predominately recognize components on the extracellular surface. In contrast, in sera made to denatured AChR, only 10–20% of the antibodies were directed against external sites. Sites recognized by most of the remainder of the antibodies could be exposed by permeabilizing the membranes with saponin, by alkaline extraction of the vesicles to remove peripheral proteins, or by a combination of these treatments. Only a small fraction (less than 20%) of the antibodies were thus directed against sites exposed upon solubilization. Competition experiments using separated subunits showed that all four subunits have buried determinants that can be exposed by the treatments above, and that α, β, and γ chains have extracellular sites that are recognized by these antibodies. These results suggest that three, and probably all four, subunits extend completely through the membrane.

It seems a natural extension of this work to use monoclonal antibodies to determine which chains and which sites are exposed on either side of the membrane. Indeed, the use of mAbs of defined specificity in combination with the technique of ultrastructural analysis and image reconstruction should lead to the definition of how different parts of the molecule are located relative to each other, to ligand binding sites, to the ion channel, and to the surrounding membrane.

5.2.3. *Different Forms of the AChR.* Antibodies are a potentially powerful tool for analyzing and distinguishing various species of the AChR present in different tissues or at different times during development. The nicotinic AChR in muscle differs pharmacologically from the nicotinic AChR in autonomic ganglia and in brain as well as from muscarinic AChRs. Little information is presently available about the immunological relation between the different AChR species. Patrick and Stallcup (1977) were able to detect cross-reacting material in a Triton-X-100 extract of PC-12, a rat pheochromocytoma cell line, by measuring the inhibition of binding of an antiserum raised against eel AChR to AChR from a muscle cell line. Moreover, they showed that the antiserum to AChR blocked carbamylcholine-induced ^{22}Na uptake by these cells. This is strong evidence for immunological cross-reaction between the neuronal AChR and the AChR from muscle and eel electric organ. The PC-12 cells also bind [^{125}I]α-BuTx, in a reaction whose pharmacological specificity is similar to that shown by sympathetic cells and by brain membranes. Curiously, however, toxin does not block ^{22}Na uptake by PC-12 cells, nor does the eel antibody recognize the component that binds [^{125}I]α-BuTx. Thus, in these cells, as in mammalian sympathetic ganglion cells (Carbonetto et al., 1978; Ravdin and Berg, 1979), the receptor for the toxin seems to be distinct from the functional AChR.

An antiserum to *Torpedo* AChR has been used to localize the AChRs in frog sympathetic ganglion cells (Marshall, 1981). Electron microscopy of ganglia that had been incubated with the receptor antibody followed by a HRP-labeled second antibody shows binding to discrete patches on the postsynaptic membrane that are just opposite active zones in the presynaptic terminals. A similar distribution of binding was seen with HRP-α-bungarotoxin; in these cells synaptic transmission is blocked by the toxin (Marshall, 1981). Thus, AChRs at neuronal synapses have a sharply restricted distribution similar to that seen at the neuromuscular junction.

The use of antibodies to distinguish between developmentally different receptor types in skeletal muscle is an example of the subtle molecular distinctions that antibodies can make. Although almost all the AChRs in normal adult muscle occur at the neuromuscular junction, AChRs in denervated adult and in developing muscles also occur in the extrajunctional membrane that extends over the entire muscle surface. The extrajunctional receptors (EJRs) differ in several of their properties from those at the junction. The differences include density of packing, metabolic turnover time, and channel open time (reviewed in Fambrough, 1979). After solubilization, the two AChRs also differ in their isoelectric points (Brockes and Hall, 1975). Biochemical comparison of the two receptor types shows them to have similar subunit compositions, and one-dimensional peptide maps of the two major subunits (corresponding to α and β) show no differences between them (Nathanson and Hall, 1979).

Initial experiments showed that an antiserum to eel AChR reacted identically to the two receptor types (Brockes and Hall, 1975), but observations by Almon and Appel (1975) suggested that there might be immunological differences between them, since serum from myasthenic patients reacted better with AChR from denervated muscle than from normal muscle. Weinberg and Hall (1979) showed that this occurred because all the determinants recognized by the myasthenic sera on normal AChR were also present on the extrajunctional AChR, but the extrajunctional AChR had additional determinants not present on the junctional receptor. Competition experiments established that extrajunctional AChRs in denervated and embryonic muscle were indistinguishable. An antiserum made to the α chain of *Torpedo* AChR also reacted better with EJRs with junctional receptors JRs, suggesting that at least one of the differences between them is on the α subunit (Lindstrom *et al.*, 1979*b*).

So far monoclonal antibodies that show absolute discrimination between the two forms of AChR as predicted from the studies of Weinberg and Hall have not been found. One mAb described by Tzartos and Lindstrom (1980) reacts about four times better with EJRs than with JRs, and may recognize a site near the unique determinant(s).

Myasthenia sera that distinguish the two forms have been used to try to relate the molecular difference between them to functional differences. During synapse formation in developing muscle, clusters of AChRs appear at sites of contact with the nerve terminals. Initially, these receptors have some of the properties of embryonic or EJRs, but during further development, they acquire the properties of receptors at adult endplates. Using a myasthenic serum that preferentially binds to

EJRs, Reiness and Hall (1981) showed that the immunologically adult JR can be detected as early as the 1st postnatal week. At this time clustering and the change in metabolic turnover time have already occurred, but the change in channel open time has not. Thus the immunological difference between the two forms is probably not related to the difference in channel open times. Because for technical reasons it was not possible to determine whether the immunologically adult form was present at earlier times, the possibility that the molecular difference is related either to clustering or to the change in turnover time remains open.

5.2.4. *Inhibition of AChR Function.* The most useful antibodies against a protein are those that block function. This is particularly true of monoclonal antibodies which bind to one or more discrete sites on a protein that in principle can be identified. Thus, it should be possible to determine which parts of a protein carry out particular functions. The AChR opens a transmembrane, cation-specific ion channel in response to the binding of ACh. These two functions of the molecule—ligand binding and channel opening—can be distinguished pharmacologically by agents that affect one but not the other. Antibodies could provide a powerful tool for identifying segments of particular polypeptide chains that carry out these separate functions.

In addition to the direct perturbation of molecular function, antibodies also offer the possibility of experimentally altering the relation of a protein to cellular processes. The binding of an antibody to a protein may affect its metabolism, the regulation of its concentration within the cell, or its relation to organelles or cytoskeletal elements. We refer to the direct effects of antibody binding on function as immediate and those that are more indirect as delayed, and consider them separately. Because the response of a cell to ACh can be affected in both ways (see below), it is important in considering an individual experiment to know the length of time that the cell has been exposed to the antibody: only effects observed within 1 hr after addition of antibody are here considered to be immediate.

5.2.4.a. *Immediate Effects.* Direct inhibition of AChR function by antibody binding has been observed frequently, but different sera seem to differ widely in their ability to inhibit. This may not be surprising, since as we have emphasized above, the AChR is a complex antigen that stimulates the production of a large variety of antibodies with differing specificities. When immunoprecipitation or antibody binding is used to compare sera, these differences are minimized since the nature of the antigenic determinants is irrelevant. When the inhibition of a particular function is examined, on the other hand, antibodies against only one or a few sites are being compared and the differences are maximized.

As might be expected these differences are largest when the effects of an antiserum to a heterologous AChR are being examined. Thus antisera to eel AChR have been consistently found to block the electrophysiological response of eel electroplax to carbamylcholine (Sugiyama *et al.*, 1973; Lindstrom *et al.*, 1976c; Penn *et al.*, 1976; Karlin *et al.*, 1978), and antisera to *Torpedo* AChR block ^{22}Na uptake by *Torpedo* vesicles (Eldefrawi *et al.*, 1979), but antisera to *Torpedo* AChR may (Penn *et al.*, 1976) or may not (Karlin *et al.*, 1978) block eel electroplax and may (Green *et al.*, 1975; Penn *et al.*, 1976) or may not (Eldefrawi *et al.*, 1979) diminish the response of vertebrate muscles to ACh. A similar phenomenon is seen when the effects of myasthenic sera on various vertebrate muscles are examined: these sera have been observed to diminish the response to ACh of human muscle (Bevan *et al.*, 1977), but to have no detectable effect on the response of frog or rat muscle (Albuquerque *et al.*, 1976).

The effects of antisera on ligand binding are also highly variable. Myasthenic sera have been reported to have no effect on the binding of α-toxins to mouse or rat diaphragm (Fulpius *et al.*, 1976; Keesey *et al.*, 1976; Albuquerque *et al.*, 1976), but to diminish binding to *Torpedo* membranes (Lefvert and Bergstrom, 1977), and different sera raised against *Torpedo* AChR vary in their ability to block the binding of ACh by *Torpedo* membranes (Sanders *et al.*, 1976; Karlin *et al.*, 1978). Ligand binding, unlike the physiological response, can be measured with solubilized receptors, thus introducing a further complexity, as the ability of a particular serum to block ligand binding to the receptor *in situ* and to the solubilized receptor may differ (Sanders *et al.*, 1976; Karlin *et al.*, 1978). One source of variability between sera may be the immunization schedule. Zurn and Fulpius (1976) have shown in one case that antibodies that block toxin binding appear late in the immunization schedule.

The variation observed between sera in their ability to block ligand binding or the electrophysiological response suggests that the antibodies responsible are a minority population and that most antibodies bind without affecting function. It is possible to make a quantitative estimate of the proportion of antibodies that block ligand binding to solubilized receptors by comparing the titer of an antiserum to receptor with and without the ligand. When this has been done, using toxin or ACh, the invariable result has been that the presence of the ligand makes little difference in the titer (Patrick and Lindstrom, 1973; Lindstrom, 1976; Karlin *et al.*, 1978; Aharonov *et al.*, 1977). Thus most of the antibodies made to solubilized receptors appear to bind at sites other than those occupied by the ligands.

An interesting exception has been observed in the case of the interaction between several myasthenic sera and rat muscle receptors (Dwyer et al., 1981). For some sera, the presence of toxin caused a large decrease in antibody binding; in one of these cases the effect was much more pronounced with EJRs than with JRs. These results suggest that at least one of the determinants that distinguish the two receptor types is near the toxin-binding site. These same authors observed that prolonged incubation with glycosidases reduced the difference between the two receptor types and reduced the ability of the antibody to inhibit toxin binding. Thus, sites of glycosylation may occur near the toxin-binding site.

The observation that a small fraction of antibodies compete with α-BuTx for binding to the AChR could be misleading if antibodies bound to sites other than the toxin-binding site also block the functional response by indirect steric or conformational changes. Such effects are presumably responsible for the results obtained by Mihovilovic and Martinez-Carrion (1979), who observed that Fab fragments reduced the rate but not the extent of α-BuTx binding to the Torpedo AChR. Since most immunizations are made with soluble AChR, it might be thought that determinants that are not normally exposed could dominate the immune response and so have no effect on function. Recently, however, Froehner (1981) showed that sera to soluble AChR recognize largely extracellular determinants. There is no doubt that antibodies can bind without affecting function. Karlin et al. (1978) showed by immunohistochemical methods that antibodies in a serum raised to Torpedo AChR could bind to eel electroplax without affecting its response to cholinergic agonists; the authors interpreted this to mean that AChR must not undergo extensive movement in the membrane during ion permeation. Antibodies in the same serum bound to Torpedo membranes without affecting either binding of neurotoxin or of ACh. These results suggest that binding of antibody to any site on the receptor is not sufficient to disturb function.

Can antibodies selectively inhibit each of the two functions of the AChR? This has not been answered for antibodies that block ligand binding, because channel function cannot be assayed independently. Evidence that antibodies can affect channel function, however, comes from studies of Heinemann et al. (1977) on the effect of antisera to Electrophorus AChR on the AChRs of a mouse cell line, BC$_3$H-1. Noise analysis showed that antibodies reduced slightly both the mean conductance of the channels and their mean open time. In addition, Karlin *et al.* (1978) have shown that an antiserum to eel AChR that does not block α-toxin binding to AChR-containing membranes causes a large reduction in the depolarization of eel electroplax produced by carbamycholine.

The ultimate answer to this question, of course, will come from the use of monoclonal antibodies. Several monoclonal antibodies have been discovered that block the binding of α-toxins. Gomez *et al.* (1979) has reported one, and James *et al.* (1980) three, cases in which binding of a mAb to the AChR can be completely blocked by nanomolar concentrations of α-BuTx. For two of these (James *et al.*, 1980) but not the others, binding to the AChR is also decreased by the cholinergic ligands, carbamylcholine, and *d*-tubocurarine, at concentrations that correspond to their known affinities for the receptor. Gomez *et al.* (1979) also have reported several mAbs whose binding to AChR is partially blocked by toxin and by low-molecular-weight agonists and antagonists; in one case, facilitation occurred. These effects could be due to a conformational change induced by the ligands that altered antibody binding. Monoclonal antibodies that bind to the channel have not yet been described, but Tzartos and Lindstrom (1981) have made a preliminary report of five antibodies that block $^{22}Na^+$ efflux from vesicles but do not affect carbachol binding.

5.2.4.b. Delayed Effects of Antibody Binding to the AChR. One important conclusion from the studies of the effects of antisera, either experimentally produced or from myasthenic patients, on the response of muscle cells to ACh, is that the immediate effects of the antisera on the AChR are in general too small to explain the large deficit in receptor function seen in muscles from immunized animals or from myasthenic patients. Two observations suggested that the deficits arise indirectly over a long period of time. First, efforts to produce the disease by passive transfer of anti-AChR immunoglobulin to mice made it clear that prolonged exposure to the antibodies was required to inhibit AChR function. Second, antisera that produced little or no effect on the response of muscle cells to ACh in the first 60 min of exposure produced dramatic effects when incubated with the cells for 24 hr. Two mechanisms to explain the delayed loss of AChR function are local cytolysis and the increased degradation of AChRs to which antibodies are bound. Both of these mechanisms are found in EAMG. As this disease has been extensively reviewed elsewhere (Lindstrom, 1980; Vincent, 1980; Lindstrom and Dau, 1979; Drachman, 1981), we give only a brief description of the course of the disease here.

The symptoms of myasthenia gravis can be induced in animals by injection with AChR in complete Freund's adjuvant. Two phases of response are seen in rats, an acute phase which occurs 8–10 days after immunization and which, if not lethal, subsides in 2–3 days. This acute phase is only seen if animals are given pertussis vaccine as an additional adjuvant and so may be a response in part to excessive adjuvant (Lindstrom and Dau, 1979). The acute response can also be induced by injection of anti-AChR into rats directly (Lindstrom et al., 1976b). In both cases there is a massive phagocytic attack of the endplates (Engel et al., 1976; Lindstrom et al., 1976b). After the injection of antibody, antibody and complement C3 are found in the synaptic cleft within 6 hr. By 24 hr fragments of membrane containing AChR can be found in the synaptic cleft, while at 48 hr macrophages enter the cleft (Engel et al., 1979). After these effects subside the endplates look structurally normal, but with reduced AChR density. This reaction does not occur if rats are depleted of the C3 component of complement (Lindstrom, 1977).

The chronic phase of the response to antibodies is also associated with a reduced level of AChR, but the mechanism is different. No phagocytes are found in the synaptic region although both antibody and complement C3 can be detected there by immunocytochemistry (Engel et al., 1977a, 1979). The mechanism of AChR loss appears to be a complement-dependent, focal lysis at the postsynaptic membrane (Toyka et al., 1977; Lennon et al., 1978; Sahashi et al., 1978), resulting in the appearance of membrane fragments containing AChR in the synaptic cleft.

The second effect of anti-AChR is to induce receptor loss by antigenic modulation. The cross-linking of surface antigens by multivalent antibodies results in their internalization and degradation by lyosomes. Such a mechanism appears to account for the disappearance of AChR from the surface after exposure to antibodies. When muscles in culture are exposed to antireceptor antibodies, derived either from immunized animals or from myasthenic sera, the degradation rate of surface AChRs is increased (Anwyl et al., 1977; Bevan et al., 1977; Appel et al., 1977; Kao and Drachman, 1977). Typically, antibodies decrease the metabolic half-life of ACh receptors about threefold. As there is no corresponding increase in AChR synthesis, this results in a net loss in AChR density, which is expressed as a decrease in sensitivity to iontophoresed ACh. The effect is not an increased turnover of all membrane proteins, since only those AChRs to which antibody is bound are degraded at the increased rate. (Drachman et al., 1978a). Antibody-induced receptor clustering can be visualized directly using fluorescent α-BuTx. Both the clustering and receptor internalization require bivalent antibodies; monovalent Fab fragments are inactive, except when they themselves are cross-bridged by a second antibody (Prives et al., 1979; Drachman et al., 1978b; Lindstrom and Einarson, 1979).

The increased rate of receptor degradation in myotubes caused by antibodies has also been observed in adult muscle cells, both in organ culture and in intact animals (Reiness et al., 1978; Heinemann et al., 1978; Merlie et al., 1979a,b). Both JRs and the EJRs that appear after denervation are affected.

The relative effectiveness of antibodies directed against specific determinants in producing these delayed effects is not known, but the increasing availability of mAbs to the AChR should quickly provide answers. MAbs are capable of reducing receptor levels in vivo after passive transfer (Lennon and Lambert, 1980; Tzartos and Lindstrom, 1980) and of enhancing the rate of AChR degradation in cultured myotubes. If cross-linking is all that is required of an antibody for it to increase degradation, then one would predict that only mAbs directed against determinants that occur more than once would be effective. Indeed, the one mAb reported by Conti-Tronconi et al. (1981) to be effective is directed against the α-subunit which is present in two copies.

Because of the importance of understanding the pathophysiology of myasthenia, most attention has centered on the particular delayed effects of antibodies that reduce surface AChR levels. Antibodies may also be useful, however, in probing the interactions of the AChR with other molecules, such as those in the cytoskeleton, or in the BL. The recent development of techniques of intracellular injection of macromolecules, for instance, makes it feasible to try to block receptor sites on the cytoplasmic side of the membrane that mediate receptor clustering or changes in other properties.

6.   ANTIBODIES TO SUBSYNAPTIC STRUCTURES

The macromolecules that form the postsynaptic density presumably are important in forming the complex folds of the postsynaptic membrane and may play a role in maintaining the high density of AChRs at the synapse. Investigation of the molecular components of the density and its associated cytoskeletal structures has barely begun. Because of the difficulty of isolating these structures intact, particularly from muscle, immunological methods are indispensable to their study.

One approach is to use antibodies to purified proteins to test by immunofluorescence for components that are likely to be part of the postsynaptic specialization. Such components should show a distribution in normal muscle that is similar to that of the AChR, should show a antigenic cross-reactivity with the AChR, should remain associated with endplates after denervation, and should not be accessible from the outside of the cell. A reservation that must be borne in mind in assessing the relative staining intensity of endplate and non-endplate regions is that the synaptic infolding causes an increase in surface in the synaptic region of about sixfold (Fambrough and Hartzell, 1972).

A number of proteins associated with cytoskeletal elements or specialized areas of cell–cell attachment have been purified and used to make specific antibodies. In addition, mAbs to cytoskeletal proteins are increasingly available. So far few of these have been tested at the neuromuscular junction. An antiserum prepared against *Aplysia* body-wall actin that in mammalian cells is specific for certain forms of cytoplasmic actin stains the neuromuscular junctions of rat muscles (Hall *et al.*, 1981). Junctions are stained in denervated muscles that lack nerve terminals and Schwann cells, and intact fibers are not stained; thus the actinlike material is presumably part of the postsynaptic density and/or underlying filaments. Because staining with the antibody is seen as early as embryonic day 20 (Fig. 4), before the subsynaptic folds are present, these results raise the possibility that a form of cytoplasmic actin plays a role in receptor clustering or stabilization.

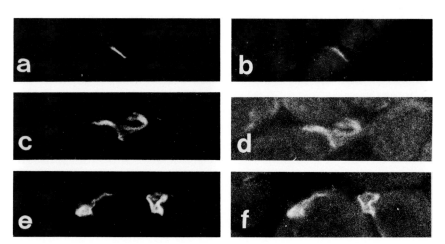

Figure 4. Antiactin binds to endplates in developing muscle. Frozen sections (6 μm) of rat diaphragm muscle viewed with rhodamine (a, c, e) and fluorescein (b, d, f) optics. (a, b) Muscle from an embryo at 18 days gestation. (c, d) Muscle from 6-day pup. (e, f) Muscle from 12-day pup. Exposures were essentially the same for each set of fluorescein prints, with minor variations for clarity. Magnification, × 750. Bar, 10 μm. (Figure reprinted from Hall *et al.*, 1981.)

Another cytoskeletal protein, vinculin, has recently been shown by immunofluorescence to be associated with patches of AChRs on myotubes in primary cultures of rat muscle (Bloch and Geiger, 1980). In these cells, AChR clusters on the ventral surface are associated with broad regions of close cell contact with the substratum. Vinculin, a protein found in cultured fibroblasts at the termination of stress fibers and at focal adhesion plaques, is associated with regions of cell–cell contact in intestinal epithelial and smooth muscle cells (Geiger, 1979). In the myotubes, some clusters also occur on the dorsal surface, and these are enriched in vinculin as well. Although not sites of substrate attachment, these could represent sites of attachment with other cells.

A mAb to tonofilament protein, which forms the intermediate filaments that are characteristic of epithelial cells, shows binding to the postsynaptic density of the neuromuscular junction that is specific by the above criteria (Burden, 1981). This antigen is restricted to the synaptic region in normal muscle, but is found associated with extrasynaptic muscle membrane after muscle denervation. Its distribution closely follows that of the AChR, although the mAb does not bind to the AChR. Another mAb, obtained after immunization with the fraction of *Torpedo* electric organ which remains after washing with salt and ionic detergent, shows a pattern of binding identical to that of the tonofilament protein (Burden, 1981). This antigen has not yet been characterized.

Another approach has been to use antisera made against peripheral proteins associated with AChR-rich membrane fragments from *Torpedo* electric organ (Froehner *et al.*, 1981). These can be removed from the membranes by an alkaline wash that does not affect the binding of cholinergic ligands nor the specific ion permeation mediated by the receptor (Neubig *et al.*, 1979; Moore *et al.*, 1979). The major component of the proteins recovered in the wash is a 43,000-dalton protein that is distinct from actin. Antisera made to extracted proteins react principally with the 43K protein and bind specifically to the innervated face of *Torpedo* electrocytes. Antibodies in the serum also bind strongly to synaptic structures in sections of normal and denervated rat muscle. Faint staining of extrasynaptic membranes was also seen (Froehner *et al.*, 1981).

It is already clear from these early results that immunological methods will be a powerful tool in unraveling the structure and the functional role of cytoskeletal elements at the neuromuscular junction. The use of mAbs will undoubtedly lead to the identification of new proteins; we look to this, and to the extension of localization studies to the ultrastructural level for future advances.

7. CONCLUSION

Antibodies can be made that specifically recognize elements of the neuromuscular junction. The antigenic elements of the neuromuscular junction fall into three classes: purified proteins such as AChR, CAT, and AChE whose synaptic function is known; proteins like actin and protein I which have been purified to homogeneity but for which a synaptic function has not yet been discovered; and synapse specific antigens which have not been purified or characterized biochemically but which are recognized by antibodies raised to subcellular elements such as synaptic vesicles, plasma membrane, or basal lamina. Since the neuromuscular junction is so small, it itself is usually unable to provide enough immunogen to raise high-titer antibodies. In general, this problem has been solved by using an alternative plentiful source of the antigen, the electric organ of fish, for example, and relying on antigenic cross-reactivity between the plentiful source and the neuromuscular junction.

Given specific antibodies, what sorts of experiments become possible? Antibodies are conventionally used as cytochemical markers, as inhibitors of function, in radioimmune assays to quantitate antigens, in purification by adsorption, in establishing the evolutionary relatedness of antigens, in studies of the biogenesis of the antigen, and in structural studies. The antibodies to neuromuscular junction elements have been used in all these ways, but obviously the function to which they are best suited depends on whether they are to pure or impure antigens, and whether the function of the antigen is known. For example, antibodies to purified molecules such as AChR and AChE have not been extensively used as markers or inhibitors since excellent alternative techniques are available. Antibodies to these molecules have been of most value in structural studies. Antibodies to molecules like actin which are more widely distributed in tissues have shown unequivocally the presence of these molecules in the synapse, and raised questions about their role in synaptic function or in maintaining synaptic structure. It is difficult to see how this information could be acquired in any other way.

Antisera which specifically stain the neuromuscular junction have also been generated using complex immunogens such as BL. These antibodies are useful in that they draw attention to molecules unique to the junction that might be missed by other techniques. It is relatively easy to determine if the corresponding antigens are postsynaptic or presynaptic or are associated with the synaptic cleft. The antibodies have also been used to delineate developmental stages of the developing or regenerating junctions and, in the case of antibodies to synaptic vesicles, to monitor synaptic activity.

It is reasonable to wonder if much is to be gained by generating antibodies to complex antigens of unknown function and unknown structure. We argue here that much is to be gained. For some questions, such as the route or routes of vesicle membrane and presynaptic plasma membrane biosynthesis and recycling, the nature of the antigen is not important, only that it be specific. When unique antigens are found by immunological techniques it is possible to purify them by conventional biochemical means or to identify them by hybridoma technology. Indeed the availability of polyclonal sera simplifies the task of designing an appropriate screening procedure for monoclonal antibodies. For example, it is useful to know if a function can be inhibited using antisera to complex antigens, before searching for an inhibitory monoclonal antibody. A valid criticism of using antibodies to identify and even purify a synapse specific antigen is that its function could still be obscure, unless the function could be assayed and the antibodies were inhibitory. Nonetheless, it is hard to believe that knowing specific molecules and their location in the synapse could do anything but facilitate our understanding of synaptic function and development.

One serendipitous consequence of raising antibodies to the components of nerve terminals has been the discovery of EAMG. Knowing that antibodies to AChR are involved in the disease state has provided powerful clues to the mechanism of autoimmune diseases in general and to myasthenia gravis and its treatment in particular. We are immediately led to wonder if antibodies to other extracellular components of the neuromuscular junction will be associated with different neuromuscular disorders. Although animals generating antibodies to synaptic cleft elements and to antigens of the presynaptic plasma membrane have so far shown no obvious neurological symptoms, the possibility of correlating disease state and synaptic antigens remains an exciting one.

It is hard to be anything but optimistic about the future of neuromuscular junction immunology. Detailed mapping of the functional regions of the AChR in its various forms should be possible as more and more monoclonal antibodies that are characterized become available. Identification of the unique antigens in the synaptic cleft and the nerve terminal should result from combination of standard biochemistry and hybridoma technology. A powerful approach here will be a boot-strapping one. For example, antibodies raised to purified synaptic vesicles have been used to purify presynaptic plasma membrane, for which no previous marker was available. The plasma membrane was then itself used as an immunogen to generate another specific antiserum. In similar ways we would expect that antibodies to unique components of the synaptic cleft could be used to partially purify the synaptic cleft material, using immunoadsorption techniques. Use of the immunoadsorbed material as an immunogen should enrich for scarce synaptic cleft specific antigens. Boot-strapping in this way should bring relatively inaccessible components of the nerve terminal within our grasp.

It is not a wild leap of the imagination to predict that soon we will have antibodies to the calcium channel, the choline and adenosine uptake sites, the calcium ATPase of the synaptic vesicle, and the elements of the synaptic cleft involved in specific synaptic recognition and regeneration, for example. We should be able to locate these antigens at the ultrastructural level and to monitor their sequence of appearance during synaptic development. Antibodies such as these can be used to recognize proteins altered during synaptic activity and can provide a quantitative assay of synaptic development. Such assays will be indispensable for unraveling the mechanisms of communication between the elements of the junction that must occur during development and during normal function in the adult.

Acknowledgments

We thank Liz Neville and Veronica Oliva for their help in preparing the manuscript. Work in the authors' laboratories was sponsored by research grants from the NIH, the NSF, and the Muscular Dystrophy Association of America.

8.   REFERENCES

Aharonov, A., Abramsky, O., Tarrab-Hazdai, R., and Fuchs, S., 1975, Humoral antibodies to acetylcholine receptor in patients with myasthenia gravis, Lancet, 2(7930) Aug. 1975, 340.

Aharonov, A., Tarrab–Hazdai, R., Silman, I., and Fuchs, S., 1977, Immunochemical studies on acetylcholine receptor from Torpedo californica, Immunochem. 14:124.

Albuquerque, E. N., Rash, J. E., Mayer, R. F., and Satterfield, J. R., 1976, An electrophysiological and morphological study of the neuromuscular junction in patients and myasthenia gravia, Exp. Neurol. 51:536.

Almon, R. R., and Appel, S. H., 1975, Interaction of myasthenic serum globulin with the acetylcholine receptor, Biochem. Biophys. Acta 393:66.

Anderson, M. J., and Cohen, M. W., 1974, Fluorescent staining of acetylcholine receptors in vertebrate skeletal muscle, J. Physiol. (London) 237:385.

Anglister, L., Leibovich, S. J., and Silman, I., 1979, Limited digestion with pepsin as a tool for studying the molecular structure of elongated forms of electric eel acetylcholinesterase, VII Meeting of the International Society for Neurochemistry, Jerusalem, Abstract, p. 196.

Anwyl, R., Appel, S. M., and Narahashi, T., 1977, Myasthenia gravis serum reduces acetylcholine sensitivity in cultured rat myotubes, *Nature (London)* **267**:262.

Appel, S. M., Almon, R. R., and Levy, N., 1975, Acetylcholine receptor antibodies in myasthenia gravis, *N. Engl. J. Med.* **293**:760.

Appel, S. M., Anwyl, R., McAdams, M. W., and Elias, S., 1977, Accelerated degradation of acetylcholine receptor from cultured rat myotubes with myasthenia gravis sera and globulins, *Proc. Natl. Acad. Sci. U.S.A.* **74**:2130.

Bartfield, D., and Fuchs, S., 1977, Immunological characterization of an irreversibly denatured acetylcholine receptor, *FEBS Lett.* **77**:214.

Bartfield, D., and Fuchs, S., 1979, Active acetylcholine receptor fragment obtained by tryptic digestion of acetylcholine receptor from *Torpedo californica, Biochem. Biophys. Res. Commun.* **89**:512.

Benda, P., Tsuji, S., Daussant, J., and Changeux, J.-P., 1970, Localization of acetylcholinesterase by immunofluorescence in eel electroplax, *Nature (London)* **225**:1149.

Berman, P. W., and Patrick, J., 1980, Experimental myasthenia gravis. A murine system, *J. Exp. Med.* **151**:204.

Bevan, S., Kullberg, R. W., and Heinemann, S. F., 1977, Human myasthenic sera reduce acetylcholine sensitivity of human muscle cells in tissue culture, *Nature (London)* **267**:263.

Bloch, R. J., and Geiger, B., 1980, The localization of acetylcholine receptor clusters in areas of cell-substrate contact in cultures of rat myotubes, *Cell* **21**:25.

Bloom, F. E., Ueda, T., Battenberg, E., and Greengard, P., 1979, Immunocytochemical localization, in synapses, at protein I, an endozenous substrate for protein kinases in mammalian brain, *Proc. Nat. Acad. Sci.* **76**:5982.

Bon, S., Vigny, M., and Massoulie, J., 1979, Asymmetric and globular forms of acetylcholinesterase in mammals and birds, *Proc. Natl. Acad. Sci. U.S.A.* **76**:2546.

Boulter, J., and Patrick, J., 1977, Purification of an acetylcholine receptor from a nonfusing muscle cell line, *Biochemistry* **16**:4900.

Bourgeois, J. P., Ryter, A., Menez, A., Fromageot, P., Boquet, P., and Changeux, J.-P., 1972, Localization of the cholinergic receptor protein in *Electrophorus* electroplax by high resolution autoradiography, *FEBS Lett.* **25**:127.

Bourgeois, J. P., Tsuji, S., Boquek, P., Pillot, J., Ryter, A., and Changeux, J. P., 1971, Localization of the cholinergic receptor protein by immunofluorescence in eel electroplay, *FEBS Lett.* **16**:92.

Brockes, J., and Hall, Z. W., 1975, Acetylcholine receptors in normal and denervated rat diaphragm muscle. II. Comparison of junctional and extrajunctional receptors, *Biochemistry* **14**:2100.

Burden, S., 1981, Monoclonal antibodies to the frog nerve–muscle synapse, in: *Monoclonal Antibodies to Neural Antigens* (R. McKay, M. Raff, and L. Reichardt, eds.), Cold Spring Harbor, N.Y., p. 247–258.

Burden, S. J., Sargent, P. B., and McMahan, U. J., 1979, Acetylcholine receptors in regenerating muscle accumulate at original synaptic sites in the absence of the nerve, *J. Cell Biol.* **82**:412.

Carbonetto, S. T., Fambrough, D. M., and Muller, K. J., 1978, Nonequivalence of α-bungarotoxin receptors and acetylcholine receptors in chick sympathetic neurons, *Proc. Natl. Acad. Sci. U.S.A.* **75**:1016.

Carlson, S. S., and Kelly, R. B., 1980, An antiserum specific for cholinergic synaptic vesicles from electric organ. *J. Cell Biol.* **87**:98.

e immun.

Immunology of the Neuromuscular Junction 41

Carlson, S. S., Wagner, J. A., Kelly, R. B., 1978, Purification of synaptic vesicles from elasmobranch electric organ and the use of biophysical criteria to demonstrate purity, *Biochemistry* **17**:1188.

Ceccarelli, B., and Hurlbut, W. P., 1980, Vesicle hypothesis of the release of Quanta of acetylcholine, *Physiol. Rev.* **60**:396.

Chao, L. P., 1975, Subunits of choline acetyltransferase, *J. Neurochem.* **25**:261.

Chao, L.-P., and Wolfgram, F., 1973, Purification and some properties of choline acetyltransferase (EC 2.3.1.6) from bovine brain, *J. Neurochem.* **20**:1075.

Claudio, T., and Raftery, M., 1977, Immunological comparison of acetylcholine receptors and their subunits from species of electric ray, *Arch. Biochem. Biophys.* **181**:484.

Conti-Tronconi, Bianca, Tzartos, S., and Lindstrom, J., 1981, Monoclonal antibodies as probes of acetylcholine receptor structure. II. Binding to native receptor, *Biochem.* **20**:2181.

Couteaux, R., and Pecot-Dechavassine, M., 1968, Particularities structurales du sarcoplasma sous-neural, *C. R. Acad. Sci.* **266**:8.

Couteaux, R., and Pecot-Dechavassine, M., 1970, Vesicules synaptiques et posches au niveau de "zone actives" de la jonction neuromusculaire, *C. R. Acad. Sci. Ser. D* **271**:2346.

Cozzari, C., and Hartman, B. K., 1980, Preparation of antibodies specific to choline acetyltransferase from bovine caudate nucleus and immunohistochemical localization of the enzyme. *Proc. Natl. Acad. Sci. U.S.A.* **77**:7453.

Daniels, M. P., and Vogel, Z., 1975, Immunoperoxidase staining of α-BuTx binding sites in muscle endplates shows distribution of acetylcholine receptors, *Nature (London)* **254**:339.

De Camilli, P., Veda, T., Bloom, F. E., Battenberg, E., and Greengard, P., 1979, Widespread distribution of protein 1 in the central of peripheral nervous system, *Proc. Natl. Acad. Sci. U.S.A.* **76**:5977.

Drachman, D. B., 1981, The biology of myasthenia gravia, *Ann. Rev. Neurobiol.* **4**:195.

Drachman, D. B., Angus, W. A., Adams, R. N., and Kao, I., 1978a, Effect of myasthenic patients' immunoglobulin on acetylcholine receptor turnover: Selectivity of degradation process, *Proc. Natl. Acad. Sci. U.S.A.* **75**:3422.

Drachman, D. B., Angus, C. W., Adams, R. N., Michelson, J. D., and Hoffman, G. J., 1978b, Myasthenic antibodies cross-link acetylcholine receptors to accelerate degradation, *N. Engl. J. Med.* **298**:1116.

Dwyer, D. S., Bradley, R. L., Furner, L., and Kemp, G. E., 1981, Immunochemical Properties of junctional and extrajunctional acetylcholine receptor, *Brain Res.* **217**:23.

Eldefrawi, M. E., Copio, D. S., Hudson, C. S., Rash, J., Mansour, N. A., Eldefrawi, A. T., and Albuquerque, E. X., 1979, Effects of antibodies to *Torpedo* acetylcholine receptor-ionic channel complex of *Torpedo* electroplax and rabbit intercostal muscle, *Exp. Neurol.* **64**:428.

Ellisman, M. H., Rash, J. E., Staehlin, A., and Porter, K. R., 1976, Studies on excitable membranes. II. A comparison of specializations at neuromuscular junctions and nonjunctional sarcolemmas of mammalian fast and slow twitch muscle fibers, *J. Cell Biol.* **68**:752.

Eng, L. F., Uyeda, C. T., Chao, L.-P., and Wolfgram, F., 1974, Antibody to bovine choline acetyltransferase and immunofluorescent localisation of the enzyme in neurones, *Nature (London)* **250**:243.

Engel, A. G., Tsujihata, M., Lambert, E. H., Lindstrom, J. M. and Lennon, V. A., 1976, Experimental autoimmune myasthenia gravis: A sequential and quantitative study of the neuromuscular junction ultrastructure and electrophysiological correlations, *J. Neurolpathol. Exp. Neurol.* **35**:569.

Engel, A. G., Lambert, E. H., and Howard, F. M., 1977a, Immune complexes (IgG and C₃) at the motor end-plate in myasthenia gravis, *Mayo Clinic Proc.* **52**:267.

Engel, A. G., Lindstrom, J. M., and Lambert, E. H., 1977b, Ultrastructure localization of the acetylcholine receptor in myasthenia gravis and in its experimental autoimmune model, *Neurology* **27**:307.

Engel, A. G., Sakakibara, H., Sahashi, K., Lindstrom, J. M., Lambert, E. H., and Lennon, V. A., 1979, Passively transferred experimental autoimmune myasthenia gravis, *Neurology* **29**:179.

Fambrough, D. M., 1979, Control of acetylcholine receptors in skeletal muscle, *Physiol. Rev.* **59**:165.

Fambrough, D. M., and Hartzell, H. C., 1972, Acetylcholine receptors: Number and distribution at neuromuscular junctions in rat diaphragm, *Science* **176**:189.

Fertuck, H. C., and Salpeter, M. M., 1974, Localization of acetylcholine receptor by ^{125}I-labelled α-bungarotoxin at mouse endplates, *Proc. Natl. Acad. Sci. U.S.A.* **71**:1376.

Froehner, S. C., 1981, Identification of exposed and buried determinants of the membrane-bound acetylcholine receptor from *Torpedo californica*, *Biochemistry* **20**:4905.

Froehner, S. C., and Rafto, S., 1979, Comparisons of the subunits of *Torpedo californica* acetylcholine receptor by peptide mapping, *Biochemistry* **18**:301.

Froehner, S. C., Reiness, C. G., and Hall, Z. W., 1977, Subunit structure of the acetylcholine receptor from denervated rat skeletal muscle, *J. Biol. Chem.* **252**:8589.

Froehner, S. C., Gulbrandsen, V., Hyman, C., Jene, A. Y., Neubig, R. R., and Cohen, J. B., 1981, Immunofluorescence localization at the mammalian neuromuscular junction of the Mr 43000 Protein of *Torpedo* postsynaptic membrane, *Proc. Natl. Acad. Sci. U.S.A.* **78**:5230.

Fulpius, B. W., Zurn, A. D., Granato, D. A., and Leder, R. M., 1976, Acetylcholine and myasthenia gravis, *Ann. N.Y. Acad. Sci.* **274**:116.

Geiger, B., 1979, A 130K protein from chicken gizzard: its location at the termini of microfilament bundles in cultured chicken cells, *Cell* **18**:193.

Glover, V. A. S., and Potter, L. T., 1971, Purification and properties of choline acetyltransferase from ox brain striate nuclei, *J. Neurochem.* **18**:571.

Goldberg, A. M., and McCaman, R. E., 1967, A quantitative microchemical study of choline acetyltransferase and acetylcholinesterase in the cerebellum of several species, *Life Sci.* **6**:1493.

Gomez, C. M., Richman, D. P., Berman, P. W., Burres, S. T., Arnason, B. G., and Fitch, F. W., 1979, Monoclonal antibodies against purified nicotinic acetylcholine receptor, *Biochem. Biophys. Res. Commun.* **88**:575.

Green, D. P., Miledi, R., and Vincent, A., 1975, Neuromuscular transmission after immunization against acetylcholine receptors, *Proc. R. Soc. London Ser. B* **189**:57.

Greenberg, A. J., Parker, K. K., and Trevor, A. J., 1977, Immunochemical studies of mammalian brain acetylcholinesterase. *J. Neurochem.* **29**:911.

Greengard, P., and De Camilli, P., 1981, Protein phosphorylation in neurons, in: *Diseases of the Motor Unit* (D. L. Schotland, ed.), Houghton Mifflin Professional Publications, Calif., in press.

Gullick, W. J., Tzartos, S., Lindstrom, J., 1981, Monoclonal antibodies as probes of acetylcholine receptor structures. I. Peptide mapping. *J. Biochem.* **20**:2173.

Gurari, D., Silman, I., and Fuchs, S., 1974, Immunochemical and enzymatic properties of the electric eel acetylcholinesterase-anti-acetylcholinesterase system, *Eur. J. Biochem.* **43**:179.

Hall, Z. W., 1973, Multiple forms of acetylcholinesterase and their distribution in endplate and non-endplate regions of rat diaphragme muscle, *J. Neurobiol.* **4**:343.

Hall, Z. W., Lubit, B. W., and Schwartz, J. H., 1981, Cytoplasmic actin in postsynaptic structures at the neuromuscular junction, *J. Cell Biol.* **90**:789.

Hartzell, H. C., and Fambrough, D. M., 1972, Acetylcholine receptors. Distribution and extrajunctional density in rat diaphragm after denervation correlated with acetylcholine sensitivity, *J. Gen. Physiol.* **60**:248.

Hebb, C., and Silver, A., 1956, Choline acetylase in the central nervous system of man and some other mammals, *J. Physiol.* **134**:718.

Heinemann, S., Bevan, S., Kullberg, R., Lindstrom, J., and Rice, J., 1977, Modulation of acetylcholine receptor by antibody against the receptor, *Proc. Natl. Acad. Sci. U.S.A.* **7**:3090.

Heinemann, S., Merlie, J., and Lindstrom, J., 1978, Modulation of acetylcholine receptor in rat diaphragm by anti-receptor sera, *Nature (London)* **274**:65, Simplified method for raising antibodies to rat dopamine beta-hydroxylase, *J. Neurochem.* **32**:1351.

Helle, K. B., Fillenz, M., Stanford, C., Pihl, K. E., and Srebro, B., 1979, A simplified method for raising antibodies to dopamine β–hydroxylase, *J. Neurochem.* **32**:1351.

Heuser, J. E., and Reese, T. S., 1979, Synaptic vesicle exocytosis captured by quick freezing, in: *The Neurosciences, Fourth Study Program,* (F. O. Schmitt and F. G. Worden, eds.), pp. 573–600, The MIT Press, Cambridge, Mass.

Heuser, J. E., and Salpeter, S., 1979, Organization of acetylcholine receptors in quick frozen, deep-etched and rotary-replicated *Torpedo* postsynaptic membrane, *J. Cell Biol.* **82**:150.

Heuser, J. E., Reese, T. S., Dennis, M. J., Jan, Y. N., Jan, L., and Evans, L., 1979, Synaptic vesicle exocytosis captured by quick freezing and correlated with quantal transmitter release, *J. Cell Biol.* **81**:275.

Hirokawa, N., and Heuser, J. E., 1980, Possible anchoring structure for the organized arrays of receptors seen at neuromuscular junctions, *J. Cell Biol.* **87**:83a.

Hooper, J. E., Carlson, S. S., and Kelly, R. B., 1980, Antibodies to synaptic vesicles purified from *Narcine* electric organ bind a subclass of mammalian nerve terminals, *J. Cell Biol.* **87**:104.

James, R. W., Kato, A. C., Rey, M.-J., and Fulpius, B. W., 1980, Monoclonal antibodies directed against the neurotransmitter binding site of nicotinic acetylcholine receptor, *FEBS Lett.* **120**:145.

Kao, I., and Drachman, D. B., 1977, Myasthnic immuniglobulin accelerates acetylcholine receptor degradation, *Science* **196**:527.

Karen-Kan, K. S., Chao, L. P., and Eng, L. F., 1978, Immunohistochemical localization of choline acetyltransferase in rabbit spinal cord and cerebellum, *Brain Res.* **146**:221.

Karlin, A., 1980, Molecular properties of nicotinic acetylcholine receptors, in: *The Cell Surface and Neuronal Function* (C. W. Cotman, G. Poste, and G. L. Nicholson, eds.), pp. 191–260, Elsevier/North-Holland. Amsterdam, New York.

Karlin, A., Holtzman, E., Valderrama, R., Damle, V., Hsu, K., and Reyes, F., 1978, Binding of antibodies to acetylcholine receptors in *Electrophorus* and *Torpedo* Electroplax membranes, *J. Cell Biol.* **76**:577.

Karnovsky, M. J., and Roots, L., 1964, A "direct-coloring" thiocholine method for cholinesterases. *J. Histochem. Cytochem.* **12**:219.

Keesey, J., Shaikh, I., Wolfgram, F., and Chao, L.-P., 1976, Studies on the ability of acetylcholine receptors to bind alpha-bungarotoxin after exposure to myasthenic serum, *Ann. N.Y. Acad. Sci.* **274**:244.

Kelly, R. B., Deutsch, J. W., Carlson, S. C., and Wagner, J. A., 1979, Biochemistry of neurotransmitter release, *Ann. Rev. Neurosci.* **2**:399.

Kimura, H., McGeer, P. L., Peng, J. H., and McGeer, E. G., 1980, Choline acetyltransferase containing neurons in rodent brain by immunohistochemistry, *Science* **208**:1057.

Klymkowsky, M. W., and Stroud, R. M., 1979, Immunospecific identification and three-dimensional structure of a membrane-bound acetylcholine receptor from *Torpedo californica*, *J. Mol. Biol.* **128**:319.

Klymkowsky, M. W., Heuser, J. E., and Stroud, R. M., 1980, Protease effects on the structure of acetylcholine receptor membranes from *Torpedo californica*, *J. Cell Biol.* **85**:823.

Labat-Robert, J., Saitoh, T., Godeau, G., Robert, L., and Changeux, J.-P., 1980, Distribution of macromolecules from the intercellular matrix in the electroplaque of *Electrophorus electricus*, *FEBS Lett.* **120**:259.

Lefvert, A. K., and Bergstrom, K., 1977, Immunoglobulins in myasthenia gravis: Effect of human lymph IgG3 and F(ab')$_2$ fragments on a cholinergic receptor preparation from *Torpedo marmorata*, *Eur. J. Clin. Invest.* **7**:115.

Lennon, V. A., and Lambert, E. H., 1980, Myasthenia gravis induced by monoclonal antibodies to acetylcholine receptors, *Nature (London)* **285**:238.

Lennon, V. A., Seybold, M. E., Lindstrom, J. M., Cochrane, C., and Ulevitch, R., 1978, Role of complement in the pathogenesis of experimental autoimmune myasthenia gravis, *J. Exp. Med.* **973**.

Lentz, T. L., Maxurkiowicz, J. E. and Rosenthal, J., 1977, Cytochemical localization of acetylcholine receptors at the neuromuscular junction by means of horse radish peroxidase-labeled α-bungarotoxin, *Brain Res.* **132**:423.

Lindstrom, J., 1976, Immunological studies of acetylcholine receptors, *J. Supramol. Struct.* **4**:389(349).

Lindstrom, J., 1977, An assay for antibodies to human acetylcholine receptor in serum from patients with myasthenia gravis, *Clin. Immunol. Immunopathol.* **7**:36.

Lindstrom, J., 1980, Biology of myasthenia gravis, *Ann. Rev. Pharmacol.* **20**:337.

Lindstrom, J., and Dau, P., 1979, Autoimmune response to acetylcholine receptors in myasthenia gravis and its animal model, *Adv. Immunol.* **27**:1.

Lindstrom, J., and Einarson, B., 1979, Antigenic modulation receptor loss in experimental autoimmune myasthenia gravis, *Muscle Nerve* **2**:173.

Lindstrom, J. M., Einarson, B. L., Lennon, V. A., and Seybold, M. E., 1976a, Pathological mechanisms in experimental autoimmune myasthenia gravis. I. Immunogenicity of syngeneic muscle acetylcholine receptor and quantitative extraction of receptor and antibody-receptor complexes from muscles of rats with experimental autoimmune myasthenia gravis, *J. Exp. Med.* **144**:726.

Lindstrom, J. M., Engel, A. G., Seybold, M. E., Lennon, V. A., and Lambert, E. H., 1976b, Pathological mechanisms in experimental autoimmune myasthenia gravis. II. Passive transfer of experimental autoimmune myasthenia gravis in rats with anti-acetylcholine receptor antibodies, *J. Exp. Med.* **144**:739.

Lindstrom, J. M., Lennon, V. A., Seybold, M. E., and Whittingham, S., 1976c, Experimental autoimmune myasthenia gravis and myasthenia gravis: Biochemical and immunochemical aspects, *Ann. N.Y. Acad. Sci.* **276**:259.

Lindstrom, J., Campbell, M., and Nave, B., 1978a, Specificities of antibodies to acetylcholine receptors, *Muscle Nerve* **1**:140.

Lindstrom, J., Einarson, B., and Merlie, J., 1978b, Immunization of rats with polypeptide chains from *Torpedo* acetylcholine receptor causes an autoimmune response to receptors in rat muscle, *Proc. Natl. Acad. Sci. U.S.A.* **75**:769.

Lindstrom, J., Merlie, J., and Yogeeswaran, Z., 1979a, Biochemical properties of acetylcholine receptor subunits from *Torpedo californica*, *Biochemistry* **18**:4465.

Lindstrom, J., Walter, B., and Einarson, B., 1979*b*, Immunochemical similarities between subunits of acetylcholine receptors from *Torpedo, Electrophorus,* and mammalian muscle, *Biochemistry* **18**:4470.

Lindstrom, J., Cooper, J., and Tzartos, S., 1980*a,* Acetylcholine receptors from *Torpedo* and *Electrophorus* have similar subunit structures, *Biochemistry* **19**:1454.

Lindstrom, J., Gullick, W., Conti-Tronconi, B., and Ellisman, M., 1980*b,* Proteolytic nicking of the acetylcholine receptor, *Biochemistry* **19**:4791.

Marshall, L. M., 1981, Synaptic localization of alpha-bungarotoxin binding which blocks nicotinic transmission at frog synaptic neurons, *Proc. Natl. Acad. Sci. U.S.A.* **78**:1948.

Marshall, L. M., Sanes, J. R., and McMahan, U. J., 1977, Reinnervation of original synaptic sites on muscle fiber basement membrane after disruption of the muscle cells, *Proc. Natl. Acad. Sci. U.S.A.* **74**:3073.

Massoulie, J., and Bon, S., 1982, The molecular forms of cholinesterase and acetylcholinesterase in vertebrates, *Ann. Rev. Neurosci.,* in press.

McMahan, U. J., Sanes, J. R., and Marshall, L. M., 1978, Cholinesterase is associated with the basal lamina at the neuromuscular junction, *Nature (London)* **271**:172.

Merlie, J. P., Changeux, J. P., and Gros, F., 1977, Acetylcholine receptor degradation measured by pulse chase labelling, *Nature (London)* **264**:74.

Merlie, J. P., Heinemann, S., and Lindstrom, J. M., 1979*a,* Acetylcholine receptor degradation in adult rat diaphragms in organ culture and the effect of anti-acetylcholine receptor antibodies, *J. Biol. Chem.* **254**:6320.

Merlie, J. P., Heinemann, S., Einarson, B., and Lindstrom, J. M., 1979*b,* Degradation of acetylcholine receptor in diaphragms of rats with experimental autoimmune myasthenia gravis, *J. Biol. Chem.* **254**:6328.

Mihovilovic, M., and Martinez-Carrion, M., 1979, Purification of high-affinity Fab fragments from experimental autoimmune myasthenia gravis rabbits and their effect on isolated acetylcholine receptors, *Biochemistry* **18**:4522.

Miljanich, G. P., Brasier, A. R., and Kelly, R. B., 1982, Partial purification of active zones of presynaptic plasma membrane by immunoadsorption, *Biophys. J.* **37**:(in press).

Miller, J. B., and Hall, Z. W., 1979, Monoclonal antibodies to the nicotinic acetylcholine receptor from rat muscle, *Soc. Neurosci. Abstr.* **5**:486.

Moore, H. P. H., Hartig, P. R., Wu, C. S., and Raftery, M. A., 1979, Rapid cation flux from *Torpedo californica* membrane vesicles: Companion of acetylcholine receptor enriched selectively extracted fractions, *Biochem. Biophys. Res. Commun.* **88**:735.

Moshly-Rosen, M., Fuchs, S., and Eshhar, Z., 1979, Monoclonal antibodies against defined determinants of acetylcholine receptor, *FEBS Lett.* **106**:389.

Nathanson, N. M., and Hall, Z. W., 1979, Subunit structure and peptide mapping of junctional and extrajunctional acetylcholine receptors from rat muscle, *Biochemistry* **15**:3392.

Neubig, R. R., Krodel, E. K., Boyd, N. D., and Cohen, J. B., 1979, Acetylcholine and local anesthetic binding to *Torpedo* nicotinic postsynaptic membranes after removal of non-receptor peptides, *Proc. Natl. Acad. Sci. U.S.A.* **76**:690.

Padykula, H. A., and Gauthier, G. F., 1970, The ultrastructure of the neuromuscular junctions of mammalian red, white and intermediate skeletal muscle fibers, *J. Cell Biol.* **46**:27.

Patrick, J., and Lindstrom, J., 1973, Autoimmune response to acetylcholine receptor, *Science* **180**:871.

Patrick, J., and Stallcup, W. B., 1977, Immunological distinction between acetylcholine receptor and the α-bungarotoxin-binding component on sympathetic neurons. *Proc. Natl. Acad. Sci. U.S.A.* **74**:4698.

Peng, H. B., 1981, Correlation of surface ACh receptor clusters with cytoplasmic structures in cultured muscle cells, *J. Cell Biol.* **87**:83a.

Peng, J. H., McGeer, P. L., Kimura, H., Sung, S. C., and McGeer, E. G., 1980, Purification and immunochemical properties of choline acetyltransferase from human brain, *Neurochem. Res.* **5**:943.

Peng, J. H., Kimura, H., McGeer, P. L., and McGeer, E. G., 1981, Anti-choline acetyltransferase fragments antigen binding (Fab) for immunohistochemistry, *Neurosci. Lett.* **21**:281.

Penn, A. S., Chang, H. W., Lovelace, R. E., Niemi, W., and Miranda, A., 1976, Antibodies to acetylcholine receptors in rabbits: Immunological and electrophysiological studies, *Ann. N.Y. Acad. Sci. U.S.A.* **274**:354.

Porter, C. W., and Barnard, E. A., 1975, The density of cholinergic receptors at the endplate postsynaptic membrane: Ultrastructural studies in two mammalian species, *J. Membr. Biol.* **20**:31.

Potter, L. T., Glover, V. A. S., and Jaelens, J. K., 1968, Choline acetyltransferase from rat brain, *J. Biol. Chem.* **243**:3684.

Prives, J., Noffman, L., Tarrab-Hazdai, R., Fuchs, S., and Amsterdam, A., 1979, Ligand induced changes in stability and distribution of acetylcholine receptors on surface membranes of muscle cells, *Life Sci.* **24**:1713.

Raftery, M. A., Hunkapiller, M. W., Strader, C. D., and Hood, L. E., 1980, Acetylcholine receptor: Complex of homologous subunits, *Science* **208**:1454.

Rash, J. E., Albuquerque, E. X., Hudson, C. S., Mayer, R. F., and Satterfield, J. R., 1976, Studies of human myasthenia gravis: Electrophysiological and ultrastructural evidence compatible with antibody attachment to the acetylcholine receptor complex, *Proc. Natl. Acad. U.S.A.* **73**:4584.

Ravdin, P. M., and Berg, D. K., 1979, Inhibition of neuronal acetylcholine sensitivity by α-toxins from *Bungarus multicinctus* venom, *Proc. Natl. Acad. Sci. U.S.A.* **76**:2072.

Reiness, C. G., and Hall, Z. W., 1981, The developmental change in immunological properties of the acetylcholine receptor in rat muscle, *Dev. Biol.* **81**:324.

Reiness, C. G., Weinberg, C. B., and Hall, Z. W., 1978, Antibody to acetylcholine receptor increases degradation of junctional and extrajunctional receptors in adult muscle, *Nature (London)* **274**:68.

Rieger, R., Benda, P., Baumann, A., and Rossier, J., 1973, Immunological studies on globular and elongated forms of electric eel acetylcholinesterase. Effects on hydrolytic enzymes, *FEBS Lett.* **32**:62.

Rossier, J., 1975, Immunohistochemical localization of choline acetylcholinesterase: Real or artifact? *Brain Res.* **98**:619.

Rossier, J., 1976, Biophysical properties of rat brain choline acetyltransferase. *J. Neurochem.* **26**:555.

Rossier, J., 1977, Choline acetyltransferase: A review with special reference to its cellular and subcellular localization, *Int. Rev. Neurobiol.* **20**:283.

Ryan, R. L., and McClure, W. O., 1979, Purification of choline acetyltransferase from rat and cow brain, *Biochemistry* **18**:5357.

Sahashi, K., Engel, A. G., Lindstrom, J. M., and Lambert, E. H., 1978, Ultrastructural localization of immune complexes (IgG and C3) at the endplate in experimental autoimmune myasthenia gravis, *J. Neuropathol. Exp. Neurol.* **37**:212.

Saito, K., Barba, R., Wu, J.-Y., Matsuda, T., Roberts, E., and Vaughn, J. E., 1974, Immunohistochemical localization of glutamate decarboxylase in rat cerebellum, *Proc. Natl. Acad. Sci. U.S.A.* **71**:269.

Sanders, D. B., Schleifer, L. S., Eldefrawi, M. E., Norcross, N. L., and Cobb, E. E., 1976, An immunologically induced defect of neuromuscular transmission in rats and rabbits, *Ann. N.Y. Acad. Sci.* **274**:319.

Sanes, J. R., and Hall, Z. W., 1979, Antibodies that bind specifically to synaptic sites on muscle fiber basal lamina, *J. Cell Biol.* **83**:357.

Sanes, J. R., Marshall, L. M., and McMahan, U. J., 1980, Reinnervation of Skeletal Muscle: Restoration of the Normal Synaptic Pattern, in: *Nerve Repair and Regeneration: Its Clinical and Experimental Basis* (D. L. Jewett and H. R. McCarroll, Jr., eds.), pp. 130–140, C. V. Mosby, St. Louis, Mo.

Sanes, J. R., 1982, Laminin, fibronectin and collagen in synaptic and extrasynaptic portions of muscle fiber basement membrane, *J. Cell Biol.*, in press.

Sanes, J. R., Carlson, S. S., Von Wedel, R., and Kelly, R. B., 1979, Antiserum specific for motor nerve terminals in skeletal muscle, *Nature (London)* **280**:403.

Sanes, J. R., Marshall, L. M., and McMahan, U. J., 1978, Reinnervation of muscle fiber basal lamina after removal of muscle fiber, *J. Cell Biol.* **78**:176.

Shorr, R. G., Dolly, J. W., and Barnard, E. A., 1978, Composition of acetylcholine receptor protein from skeletal muscle, *Nature (London)* **274**:283.

Shuster, L., and O'Toole, C., 1974, Inactivation of choline acetyltransferases by an antiserum to the enzyme from mouse brain, *Life Sci.* **15**:645.

Singh, V. K., and McGeer, P., 1974, Cross-immunity of antibodies to human choline acetyltransferase in various vertebrate species, *Brain. Res.* **82**:356.

Stanley, E. F., and Drachman, D. B., 1978, Effect of myasthenic immunoglobulin on acetylcholine receptors of intact mammalian neuromuscular junctions, *Science* **200**:1285.

Strader, C. B., Revel, J.-P., and Raftery, M. A., 1979, Demonstration of the transmembrane nature of the acetylcholine receptor by labeling with anti-receptor antibodies, *J. Cell Biol.* **83**:499.

Sternberger, L. A., 1974, *Immunochemistry*, Prentice-Hall, Englewood Cliffs, N.J.

Sugiyama, H., Benda, P., Meunier, J. C., and Changeux, J.-P., 1973, Immunological characterization of the cholinergic receptor protein from *Electrophorus electricus*, *FEBS Lett.* **35**:124.

Tarrab-Hazdai, R., Geiger, B., Fuchs, S., and Amsterdam, A., 1978, Localization of acetylcholine receptor in excitable membrane from the electric organ of *Torpedo*: Evidence for exposure of receptor antigenic sites on both sides of the membrane, *Proc. Natl. Acad. Sci. U.S.A.* **75**:2497.

Toyka, K. V., Daniel, M. D., Drachman, B., Griffin, D. E., Pestronk, A., Winkelstein, J. A., Fischbeck, K. H., and Kao, I., 1977, Myasthenia gravis, Study of humoral immune mechanisms by passive transfer to mice, *N. Engl. J. Med.* **296**:135.

Tsuji, S., Rieger, F., Peltre, E., Massoulie, J., and Benda, P., 1972, Acetylcholinesterase du muscle, de la moelle épiniere et du cerveau de gymnote, *J. Neurochem.* **19**:989.

Tzartos, S. J., and Lindstrom, J. M., 1980, Monoclonal antibodies used to probe acetylcholine receptor structure: Localization of the main immunogenic region and detection of similarities between subunits, *Proc. Natl. Acad. Sci. U.S.A.* **77**:755.

Tzartos, S., and Lindstrom, J., 1981, Production and characterization of monoclonal antibodies for use as probes of acetylcholine receptors, in press.

Vigny, M., Koenig, J., and Rieger, F., 1976, The motor end–plate specific form of acetylcholinesterase: Appearance during embryogenesis and reinnervation of rat muscle, *J. Neurochem.* **27**:1347.

Vincent, A., 1980, Immunology of acetylcholine receptors in relation to myasthenia gravis, *Physiol. Rev.* **60**:756.

Wagner, J. A., and Kelly, R. B., 1979, Topological organization of proteins in an intracellular secretory organelle: The synaptic vesicle, *Proc. Natl. Acad. Sci. U.S.A.* **76:**4126.

Wedel, R. J. von, Carlson, S. S., and Kelly, R. B., 1981, Transfer of synaptic vesicle antigens to the presynaptic plasma membrane during exocytosis, *Proc. Natl. Acad. Sci. U.S.A.* **78:**1014.

Weinberg, G. B., and Hall, Z. W., 1979, Antibodies from patients with myasthenia gravis recognize determinants unique to extrajunctional acetylcholine receptors, *Proc. Natl. Acad. U.S.A.* **76:**504.

Weinberg, C. B., Reiness, C. G., and Hall, Z. W., 1981a, Topographical segregation old and new acetylcholine receptors at developing ectopic endplates in adult rat muscle, *J. Cell Biol.* **88:**215.

Weinberg, C. B., Sanes, J. R., and Hall, Z. W., 1981b, Formation of neuromuscular junctions in adult rats: Accumulation of acetylcholine receptors, acetylcholinesterase, and components of synaptic basal lamina, *Dev. Biol.* **84:**255.

Wenthold, R. L., and Mahler, H. R., 1975, Purification of rat brain choline acetyltransferase and an estimation of its half-life, *J. Neurochem.* **24:**963.

White, H. L., and Wu, J. C., 1973, Separation of apparent multiple forms of human brain choline acetyltransferase by isoelectric focusing, *J. Neurochem.* **21:**939.

Williams, R. M., 1969, Antibodies to acetylcholinesterase, *Proc. Natl. Acad. U.S.A.* **62:**1175.

Zurn, A. D., and Fulpius, B. W., 1976, Accessibility to antibodies of acetylcholine receptors in the neuromuscular junction, *Clin. Exp. Immunol.* **24:**9.

2

Monoclonal Antibodies to Skeletal Muscle Cell Surface

DOUGLAS M. FAMBROUGH, ELLEN K. BAYNE, JOHN M. GARDNER, M. JOHN ANDERSON, ERIC WAKSHULL, and RICHARD L. ROTUNDO

1. INTRODUCTION

About half of the mass of a vertebrate's body is muscle tissue, of which the principal cell is the muscle fiber: an extremely long, multinucleate cell which has a regionally specialized surface for interaction with tendons, for propagation of action potentials, and for reception of chemical signals from motor neurons. The intimate relation between motor neuron and muscle fiber has been of special importance to neurobiologists. Studies of the neuromuscular junction have provided fundamental information about synaptic communication. Furthermore, evidence of long-term trophic interactions between muscle fibers and motor neurons has been important for the development of ideas about the plasticity and stability of neuronal connections.

Our focus of research has been upon those mechanisms which control the expression and organization of cell surface properties during muscle development and synaptogenesis. Acetylcholine receptors (AChRs) and acetylcholinesterase (AChE) of skeletal muscle participate in these

DOUGLAS M. FAMBROUGH, ELLEN K. BAYNE, JOHN M. GARDNER, M. JOHN ANDERSON, ERIC WAKSHULL, and RICHARD L. ROTUNDO   Department of Embryology, Carnegie Institution of Washington, Baltimore, Md. 21210.

phenomena, and the availability of highly specific and strongly binding probes (the alpha neurotoxins and their derivatives for AChR, organophosphates for AChE) has facilitated research in this area. Studies of AChRs and AChE have yielded hints that the muscle cell surface is both complex and well ordered. To gain a more encompassing view of the order and complexity of the muscle cell surface we need to examine other muscle surface proteins. However, until recently, specific probes for them have not been available. Monoclonal antibody techniques now provide a means of generating specific probes for all surface proteins. In this chapter, one of our aims is to describe the course of our research before the advent of monoclonal antibody technology and to point out ways in which immunological techniques can extend the scope of our investigation. Another aim is to describe some elements of technique which we have found especially useful in preparing monoclonal antibodies. Finally, we report some preliminary observations which come from our current studies on the organization of the muscle cell surface. These observations increasingly lead us to view the cell surface as an intricate multilayered structure whose elaboration during development provides a fascinating puzzle.

2.   REGULATION OF ACETYLCHOLINE RECEPTORS

It has long been known that the number and distribution of AChRs reflect the developmental and physiological state of muscle cells. Electrophysiological studies of cholinergic sensitivity in embryonic, adult, and denervated skeletal muscle have provided the foundation upon which further analyses have rested. The discovery of α-bungarotoxin has allowed more direct and quantitative descriptions of receptor distributions (reviewed in Fambrough, 1979). The adult neuromuscular junction is now known to contain about 3×10^7 ACh binding sites, probably two sites per receptor molecule, packed into the postsynaptic membrane at about 2×10^4 sites per μm^2. The adjacent perijunctional plasma membrane has about three orders of magnitude fewer sites, and more distant extrajunctional plasma membrane shows virtually no sites at all. The large increase in chemosensitivity which occurs after denervation of adult muscle is due to a widespread appearance of extrajunctional AChRs, which may accumulate to a packing density of about 500 sites per μm^2. Because of the disproportionate area of extrajunctional plasma membrane compared to endplate, the total number of AChR attained after denervation far exceeds the number of junctional receptors.

In order to understand the mechanisms which regulate these striking changes in AChR distribution, we have devoted much of our time to the study of AChR metabolism. For these studies tissue-cultured muscle has turned out to be of greatest utility, and it has been possible to confirm or reproduce many of our findings by using organ-cultured adult muscle. Figure 1 illustrates several important features of AChR metabolism. In cultured embryonic skeletal muscle about 75% of the AChRs are in the plasma membrane. Their distribution can be visualized by light-microscope autoradiography after exposure to iodinated α-bungarotoxin. As illustrated in Fig. 2 for rat skeletal muscle, toxin binding sites are distributed over the entire myotube surface, with several discrete regions having a much higher density of binding sites. The proportions of AChRs which occur in these dense clusters apparently change during myogenesis and can be experimentally manipulated by varying culture conditions. However, the kinetics of production and turnover of AChR sites appear to be independent of such changes in spatial distribution.

The kinetics of AChR production, incorporation into plasma membrane, and turnover have been measured most directly by labeling cultured muscle cells with heavy-isotope-containing amino acids (De-

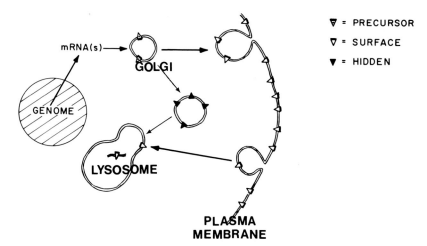

Figure 1. Schematic representation of the metabolism of AchRs. The diagram represents a cross-section through a part of a cell with membrane profiles symbolized by double lines and the AChRs by triangles with the ACh binding sites on the thickened sides. Hidden sites are represented by black triangles located in unidentified intracellular membranes. Newly synthesized sites destined for exposure on the cell surface (and contributing to the hidden receptor pool) are symbolized by triangles containing a dot. (Modified from Devreotes and Fambrough, 1976b.)

vreotes and Fambrough, 1976*a,b*; Devreotes *et al.*, 1977; Gardner and Fambrough, 1979). Incorporation of the isotopically labeled amino acids into AChRs results in a substantial change in the buoyant density of the AChR, making it possible to separate labeled from unlabeled receptors and quantify the respective receptor populations. Such experiments indicate that within 15 min of switching culture media to one containing heavy amino acids, full-sized AChR units composed of heavy aminoacyl residues have been assembled within the myotubes. The intracellular pool of these newly made receptors becomes fully labeled after about 3 hr. Only then do heavy receptors begin to constitute the major portion of AChRs appearing in the plasma membrane (shown in Fig. 3). The intracellular pool of newly synthesized receptors has been shown by quantitative electron microscope (EM) autoradiography to reside mostly in the Golgi apparatus (Fig. 4).

Pulse-chase experiments with heavy amino acids indicate that the turnover rates are similar for heavy and normal AChRs. The kinetics of turnover can be described as a first-order exponential process with a half-time of about 17 hr (Fig. 5). This turnover rate is not changed by saturation of receptor sites with either agonist (carbachol) or antagonist (*d*-tubocurare) (Gardner and Fambrough, 1979).

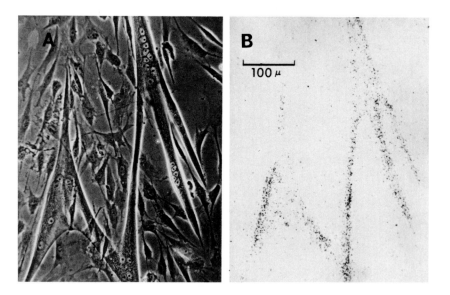

Figure 2. Autoradiograph of tissue-cultured rat skeletal muscle together with phase micrograph of the same field, AChR sites labeled with [^{125}I]α-bungarotoxin. Note nonuniform distribution of receptor sites on myotube and lack of binding sites on fibroblastic cells. (From Hartzell and Fambrough, 1973.)

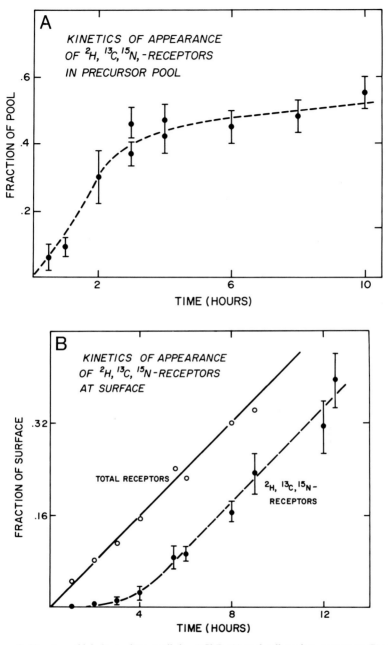

Figure 3. Kinetics of labeling of intracellular AChR (A) and cell surface receptors (B) with heavy-isotopically labeled amino acids provided in the medium of tissue-cultured chick skeletal muscle. Introduction of heavy amino acids beginning at time zero and continuing through the experimental period. Note rapid labeling of intracellular AChR sites due to *de novo* synthesis and labeling of muscle surface AChR sites only after a lag period of several hours. (From Devreotes *et al.*, 1977.)

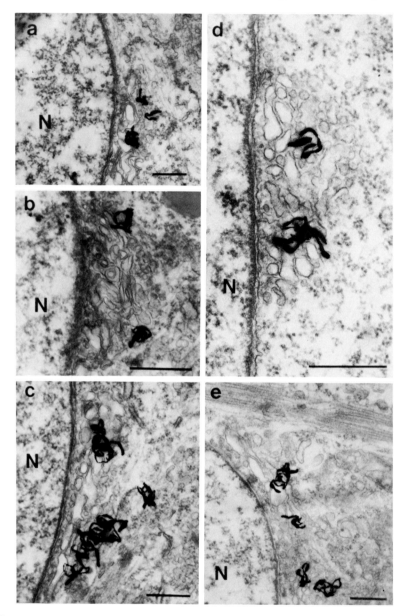

Figure 4. EM autoradiographs of sections of tissue-cultured chick myotubes after fixation, permeabilization, and saturation of intracellular AChR sites with ^{125}I-labeled α-bungarotoxin. Note association of silver grains with the Golgi apparatus. N (nucleus). Magnification bars represent 0.5 μm. (Unpublished micrographs from the study of Fambrough and Devreotes, 1978.)

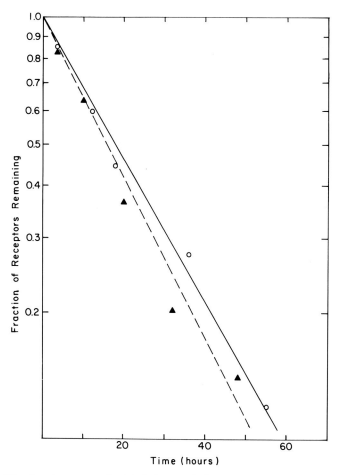

Figure 5. Kinetics of turnover of unlabeled (○) and of heavy-amino-acid-labeled (▲) AChRs in tissue-cultured chick myotubes. (From Gardner and Fambrough, 1979.)

By labeling receptors with iodinated α-bungarotoxin and following the degradation of the labeled toxin, a fair approximation of the true AChR turnover rate can be obtained. EM autoradiographic analysis (Fambrough *et al.*, 1978) has shown that toxin–receptor complexes are transported from the cell surface to secondary lysosomes, where degradation occurs (unless lysosomal hydrolases are blocked) (Fig. 6). The strategy of metabolic labeling with dense amino acids does not require purification of the AChR, and the heavy-labeled receptor molecules function normally. However, this procedure is both expensive and la-

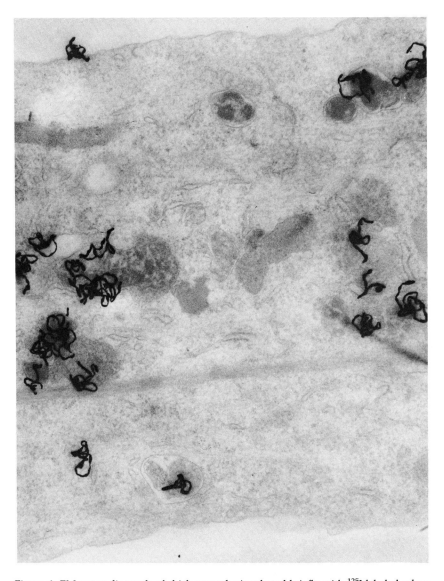

Figure 6. EM autoradiograph of chick myotube incubated briefly with ^{125}I-labeled α-bungarotoxin to saturate cell surface AChRs and then incubated in the absence of bungarotoxin for 6 hr. Myotube had been cultured in the presence of trypan blue overnight before labeling, so that degradation of toxin–receptor complexes was inhibited. Note heavy accumulation of silver grains over distended secondary lysosomes. Quantitation of autoradiographs indicated that 21.7% of silver grains were over lysosomal profiles.

borious. We expect that with the aid of monoclonal antibodies to other surface components it will be possible to use more conventional radioisotopic labeling of cells in standard pulse and pulse-chase labeling regimes, followed by purification of antigenic entities, to obtain synthetic and turnover rates for other membrane components.

Regulation of AChR number could conceivably be accomplished either by changing the rate of biosynthesis or degradation. In fact, each possible form of regulation has been documented for AChRs. Receptor levels increase during development when new receptor biosynthesis commences and also following denervation. In each case accelerated AChR production has been documented by direct metabolic labeling of receptors. Decreases in receptor number occur due to a diminished rate of production during (1) culture of embryonic muscle in the presence of carbachol (Noble *et al.*, 1978; Gardner and Fambrough, 1979), (2) electrical stimulation of denervated muscle (Lomo and Westgaard, 1975; Reiness and Hall, 1977; Linden and Fambrough, 1979), and (3) following innervation (Burden, 1977). A decrease in AChR number occurs in the disease myasthenia gravis (Fambrough *et al.*, 1973), as well as in cultured muscle exposed to immunoglobulins from myasthenic patients (Appel *et al.*, 1977; Heinemann *et al.*, 1977; Kao and Drachman, 1977). This change has been shown to result from an increase in the rate of receptor degradation. Conversely, degradation is very slow for receptors at mature neuromuscular junctions (Berg and Hall, 1975; Chang and Huang, 1975; Loring and Salpeter, 1980).

3. SKELETAL MUSCLE ACETYLCHOLINESTERASES

The analysis of the AChEs of skeletal muscle turned out to be a more complex matter than the analysis of AChR metabolism because of two added variables. First, the AChEs are a family of molecular forms whose relationships are only partially understood (Massoulie *et al.*, 1980). Second, both membrane-associated and secreted, soluble AChEs occur in skeletal muscle (Rotundo and Fambrough, 1980a). While there is no ligand equivalent to α-bungarotoxin for study of the AChEs, it has been possible to use a sensitive enzymatic assay (which provides values of activity which are proportional to the number of enzymatic sites) and also the irreversible inhibitor diisopropylfluorophosphate. Figure 7 summarizes several elements of AChE metabolism which occur in tissue-cultured chick skeletal muscle.

These cells make primarily dimeric and tetrameric forms of AChE. Most of the dimeric form is secreted from the cells about 2–3 hr after

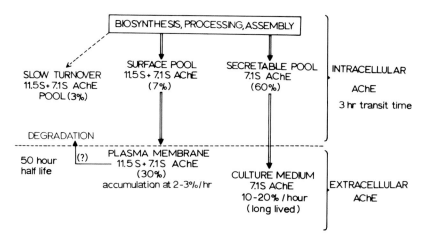

Figure 7. Schematic diagram of metabolism and distribution of AChE in tissue-cultured chick skeletal muscle. (From Rotundo *et al.*, 1980.)

biosynthesis and accumulates in the culture medium (Fig. 8B). This secretory AChE is made in relatively large amounts compared to membrane-associated AChE or AChRs. Its intracellular pool size is thus large, and about 60% of cell-associated AChE is composed of intracellular dimeric molecules synthesized within the past 3 hr. The remaining AChE is associated with the cell surface and appears to be an integral membrane protein oriented so that the enzymatic sites face outward. Renewal of membrane AChE resembles the renewal of cell surface AChRs. There is, for example, a small intracellular pool of newly synthesized molecules which, several hours after biosynthesis, become exposed on the surface. Furthermore, the turnover of the cell surface AChE also involves an energy-dependent uptake mechanism and presumably degradation within lysosomes.

The emptying and filling of the intracellular pool of secretory AChE can be observed quite easily by use of the following protocol. First, all cellular AChE is irreversibly inhibited with DFP (which readily penetrates membranes). The subsequent regeneration of the intracellular AChE can be assessed by solubilizing cells and assaying for AChE activity (Fig. 8A). The transfer of this newly made secretory AChE to the medium can be followed by labeling it with [³H]DFP and observing the near-quantitative transfer of isotope. Alternatively the enzyme loss from the cells can be measured during inhibition of further protein synthesis by cycloheximide. The secretion process is energy dependent and quite temperature sensitive, as is the transfer of AChRs from the intracellular pool to the surface.

Several aspects of AChE secretion remind one of corresponding events in AChR metabolism (Rotundo and Fambrough, 1980b). Immediately after biosynthesis both molecules occur in intracellular pools. In these pools the molecules seem to be sequestered in membrane-bound structures, for even in homogenates of muscle the enzymatic and receptor sites remain sequestered until detergent is added. The kinetics of filling and emptying of intracellular pools in both cases suggest a fairly uniform 2- to 3-hr residence time for newly synthesized molecules before their appearance at the cell surface. The sensitivity of the intra-

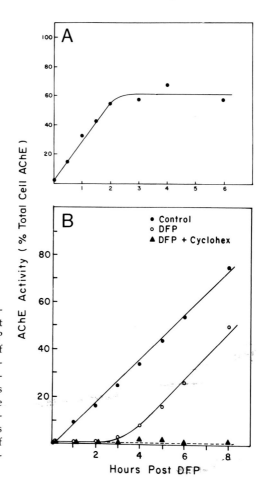

Figure 8. Kinetics of refilling of intracellular pools of AChE treatment of chick muscle cultures after DFP (A) and kinetics of resumption of AChE secretion (B). Refilling of intracellular pool is rapid, whereas repopulation of cell surface requires several days (data not shown). Note lag of several hours before resumption of secretion. Compare kinetics of production and exteriorization of AChR sites in Fig. 3. (Data from Rotundo and Fambrough, 1980a.)

cellular transport processes to colchicine and ionophores and the sensitivity of the biosynthesis-transport mechanisms to inhibitions of protein synthesis and glycosylation, seem to be identical. Likewise, the energy dependence and temperature sensitivity of the processes are quite similar. These similarities suggest further questions about membrane and secretory protein metabolism. Are the plasma membrane and secretory proteins moving together through the biosynthesis-transport process? Are they cotransported to the cell surface, perhaps in a common carrier vesicle? Might all muscle secretory proteins be produced and transported to the cell surface on the same schedule? Are coated vesicles involved in these transport processes?

The integral plasma membrane AChE led us to discover that there is not a common turnover rate for all integral plasma membrane proteins of cultured myotubes. The turnover rate of AChE was estimated by selectively labeling the cell surface with [^{3}H]DFP and then measuring the time course of degradation of labeled protein to low-molecular-weight material. To our surprise, the AChE turnover rate was three times slower than that of the AChR (Fig. 9). Less direct experiments supported this finding. For example, AChR turnover continues in the presence of tunicamycin, resulting over a few days in the loss of most cell surface AChRs. In parallel experiments we found that the cell surface AChE level declined very slowly in the presence of tunicamycin. These results indicate that the number of molecules of each plasma membrane protein may be controlled by the setting of degradation rates as well as biosynthetic rates. It would be interesting to test this hypothesis by examining the turnover of several more integral membrane proteins of skeletal muscle. We also would like to explore further the mechanism of turnover.

To summarize our work on AChRs and the AChEs, there is now a rough description of the events in the life history of each of these molecules in cultured chick skeletal muscle. Similarities in some aspects of these life histories have led us to pose a number of testable hypotheses. The plasma membrane proteins and the secretory proteins of skeletal muscle may follow a common intracellular pathway from biosynthesis to exposure at the cell surface. Secretory and plasma membrane proteins may even be transported together in vesicular structures such as coated vesicles. It may be that all of the major secretory proteins are packaged together for secretion and thus might display identical kinetics of production and secretion. Each integral membrane protein may have a unique turnover rate, although the mechanism of turnover may be general.

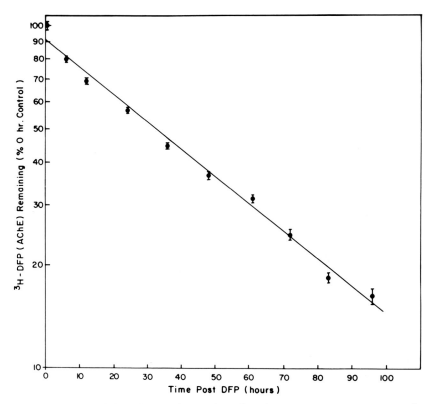

Figure 9. Kinetics of degradation of myotube cell surface AChE after labeling with [³H]-DFP. (From Rotundo and Fambrough, 1980a.)

Reflecting on studies of the AChR and AChE, one must conclude that the availability of highly specific probes and sensitive assays for specific membrane and secretory molecules was essential. Thus, in order to extend our studies to the analysis of other membrane and secretory components a new set of tools was needed. Among the possibilities, monoclonal antibodies seem to offer the largest number of useful features and highest probability of *general* utility.

4. MONOCLONAL ANTIBODIES

Monoclonal antibody technology affords the opportunity, in principle, to generate specific probes which can define each cell surface component (Kohler and Milstein, 1975; Galfre *et al.*, 1977). Such probes should also allow one to purify each component, determine which cells possess it, and in some cases determine its function. In following this experimental strategy, we have produced a number of hybridoma cell lines which secrete antibodies targeted to antigens on the muscle cell surface. The antigens defined by these probes include both integral membrane proteins and peripheral surface proteins. This collection of monoclonal antibodies has allowed us to obtain a much more complete view of the organization of the muscle cell surface and its development. With antibodies to specific integral membrane proteins we are working toward a more complete description of membrane protein turnover rates. Answering the question concerning the relation between secretion and membrane biogenesis is facilitated by monoclonal antibodies to a variety of muscle membrane and secretory proteins. As it turns out, many of the secreted proteins become incorporated into the extracellular matrix: basal lamina and more distal elements of the extracellular material. Monoclonal antibodies to these components provide us with means to study the development and organization of the extracellular matrix. While application of these immunological studies is still at an early stage, they already provide evidence which suggests that interactions may occur between components of the extracellular matrix and one integral membrane protein, the AChR.

4.1. *Monoclonal Antibody Techniques*

We have generated hybridoma cell lines using mice immunized with a variety of antigens ranging from crude preparations of *Xenopus* and chick embryo muscle to affinity purified proteins. Suspensions of the antigens in PBS were emulsified with complete Freund's adjuvant and injected into the peritoneal cavity of BALB/c mice. Approximately 1 month later the mice received a boost of the same antigen, without adjuvant or with incomplete adjuvant. After an additional 3–4 days the spleens were removed from the immunized mice and shredded and the resulting cell suspensions fused with Sp 2/0 mouse myeloma cells, using polyethylene glycol 1000. The details of the fusion protocol were similar to those described by Kennett *et al.* (1978). The myeloma line is a variant of the parent Sp 2 cell line, selected for its inability to either synthesize immunoglobulin or grow in the presence of HAT medium. To limit the tendency of the more rapidly growing hybrid cell colonies to displace all others, the cell mixture from each fusion was usually divided into 48 separate culture wells.

Approximately 1 week after fusion, substantial colonies of hybridoma cells were visible in many of the resulting cultures. At this stage a variety of immunochemical and immunocytochemical procedures were used to determine which cultures were secreting useful antibody (Fig. 10). These procedures will be described in greater detail below. Once the culture wells producing useful antibody had been identified, the cells were replated at clonal densities in soft (0.3%) agar onto a layer of 0.5% agar. In this procedure Dulbecco's minimal essential medium containing 20% fetal calf serum was used as culture medium. Cloning efficiency has proved to be very sensitive to variations between different batches of commercially prepared serum.

After approximately a week the soft agar cultures contained numerous small colonies, each representing a single hybridoma clone. These were covered with an additional layer of agar medium supplemented with antiserum specific for either mouse Fab, IgG, or IgM. This procedure resulted in the formation of precipitin disks around antibody-secreting colonies and thus permitted the selection of clones with high rates of antibody secretion and/or specific antibody isotype (Fig. 11). Such individual clones were isolated, grown in liquid medium, and reassayed. Many of the hybridomas were cloned two or three times in soft agar to insure monoclonal derivation. Immunochemical and immunocytochemical tests of the conditioned medium from cloned cultures confirmed that the cell lines were producing the same antibody species chosen in the initial screens.

In order to generate large amounts of monoclonal antibody, hybridoma cells were injected into the peritoneal cavity of BALB/c mice and grown as ascites tumors. Ascites fluid from several such mice was pooled and fractionated to isolate either IgG or IgM. This involved ammonium sulfate precipitation followed by chromatography on either DEAE-cellulose for IgG-secreting lines, or gel filtration on Ultragel AcA 22 for IgM (Fig. 12). The resulting preparations have been estimated to contain greater than 80% purified monoclonal antibody at concentrations up to approximately 2 mg/ml. As expected, such antibody preparations retain the specificity evidenced by the more dilute products (approximately three orders of magnitude more dilute) in the supernatants of hybridoma conditioned medium.

4.2. Monoclonal Antibodies Directed Against Plasma Membrane Proteins

One of the principle reasons we turned to monoclonal antibody technology was to obtain specific ligands which would define muscle

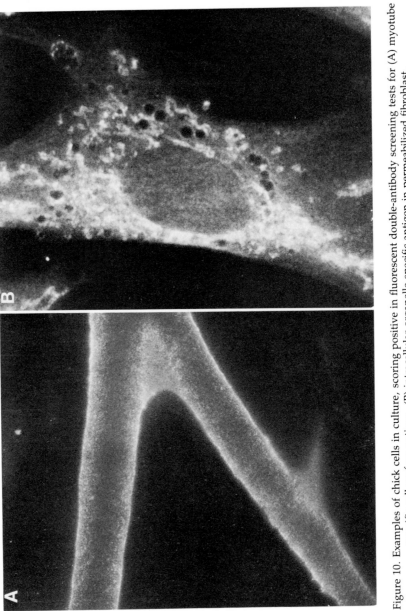

Figure 10. Examples of chick cells in culture, scoring positive in fluorescent double-antibody screening tests for (A) myotube specific cell surface antigen, (B) intracellular organelle-specific antigen in permeabilized fibroblast.

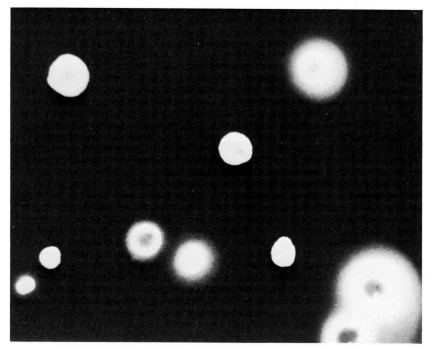

Figure 11. Hybridoma clones in agar after overlay of rabbit anti-mouse IgG. Note precipitin disks over some clones, while other clones show none. Such overlays indicate that a large number of nonsecretor variants arise from precloned, useful hybridomas. This suggests that repeated cloning may be required for maintenance of high secretion if hybridomas are kept as growing cell cultures.

plasma membrane proteins. We could then determine the turnover rates of these proteins and obtain a more complete answer to the question whether the turnover rate of each muscle plasma membrane protein is unique. Of the antibodies we have thus far produced, approximately half are targeted against membrane antigens. Our initial studies have focused on identification of the antigens recognized and on characterization of antigen distribution in terms of both cellular specificities and changes during muscle development. Such preliminary studies provide the basis for later analysis of turnover rates. They also provide some insight into the dynamics of muscle membrane development. In addition they are useful for illustrating several technical points about the use of monoclonal antibodies.

During myogenesis mononucleated myoblasts associate and fuse to form multinucleated cells called myotubes. It is clear that wholesale production of some characteristic muscle proteins begins at about the

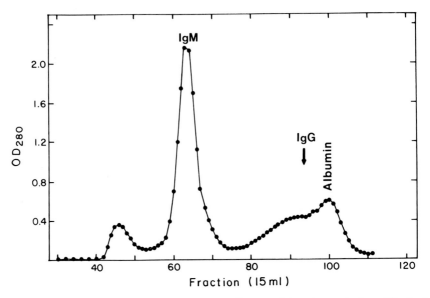

Figure 12. Elution profile of 50%-ammonium-sulfate-precipitated protein from 30 ml of hybridoma ascites fluid after resolubilization and gel filtration on Ultragel AcA 22 (LKB Instrument Co.). Note high peak of IgM eluting behind void volume peak. Column size 5 × 85 cm. Elution with borate-buffered saline at a flow rate of about 45 ml/hr. Fraction size 15 ml.

time the cells become fusion-competent. At least one membrane protein the AChR, appears as a functional entity at this time (Fambrough and Rash, 1971). Using monoclonal antibodies, we have identified a number of myogenic cell antigens (some muscle-specific, some not). Some of these antigens remain at a similar concentration in the plasma membranes of myogenic cells as they proceed through myogenesis to become mature muscle fibers. Others increase or decrease markedly (but not synchronously) during myogenesis. The fact that it is not possible to generalize about the behavior of muscle membrane antigens during development is presumably an indication that the developmental process involves asynchronous expression and repression of components.

One myogenic cell surface antigen (defined by monoclonal antibody from hybridoma #6) disappears rapidly after formation of myotubes. The antigen is also present on fibroblasts. Both fibroblasts and myoblasts, in fact, can be eliminated from myogenic cell cultures by treatment with #6 IgM and guinea pig complement, which together cause lysis of the antigen-bearing cells. After this "deep six" treatment, the remaining myotubes can be maintained in culture as a pure population (Fig. 13). Such purified myotube cultures are of great utility. They have allowed us to define which secretory proteins are synthesized by myotubes, and should permit us to investigate the properties and metabolism of myotube surface components which are shared by the other cell types present in primary muscle cultures.

Another aspect of #6 hybridoma deserves comment. In the original screening assay to detect hybridomas secreting antibody against exposed antigens in myogenic cell cultures (a binding assay using iodinated second antibody), the signal-to-background ratios for different antibodies has ranged from less than 2 to 50 or more. Hybridoma #6 was originally selected as an example whose antibody bound to a relatively rare antigen in the cultures (signal-to-background less than 2). This low signal is characteristic of binding assays even using the purified #6 IgM and is due to few antigenic sites rather than rapid dissociation of antibody. The points to be made are that (1) there is the possibility of biasing results in some unpredictable way by selecting only antibodies which recognize abundant antigens, (2) a small number of bound IgMs can carry out effective complement-mediated cytotoxicity, and (3) the utility of a monoclonal antibody may derive from one of its characteristics which was not part of the original selection scheme.

Another muscle plasma membrane antigen we have selected for immediate study (defined by monoclonal antibody C3/1) is present on both myoblasts and myotubes. It increases in abundance after cell fusion (Fig. 14) and then virtually disappears during maturation of muscle fibers. In the adult chicken, the antigen appears to be present (after staining with fluorescent or HRP-labeled IgG) primarily as a component of the satellite cells (Fig. 15). We have succeeded in purifying this antigen from tissue cultured prefusion cells after metabolic labeling with [35S] methionine. As a detergent-solubilized protein, this antigen appears to be composed of a single-size polypeptide with an approximate molecular mass of 38,000 daltons (Fig. 16).

The example of C3/1 antigen illustrates many of the criteria we have used to determine which antigens are integral plasma membrane proteins. It is a trypsin- and heat-sensitive antigen exposed on live cells and not detectable in extracellular areas of myogenic cell cultures. After exposure to fluorescent antibody the antigen appears clustered into small spots on the cells. The antigen is soluble in detergent but not in 2M NaCl or 5 mM EDTA solutions. Another class of antigens is exposed on living myogenic cells but also occurs to some extent in cell-free regions of tissue cultures and often appears to extend into acellular areas of

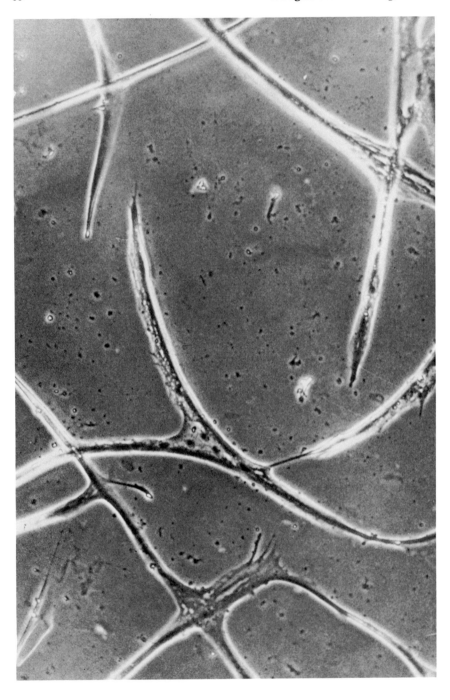

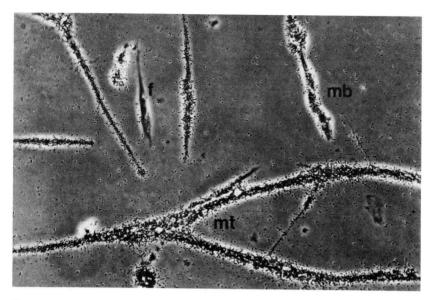

Figure 14. Light-microscope autoradiograph of chick muscle culture after labeling of binding sites to saturation with ^{125}I-labeled monoclonal antibody C3/1. Note heavy labeling of myoblasts (mb) and myotube (mt) without significant labeling of fibroblast (f).

adult skeletal muscle sections. These antigens often occur in fibrils, nets, and patches and generally are not extracted with Triton-X-100-containing solution.

An additional aspect of C3/1 which typifies a number of our monoclonal antibodies is that the antibody binds specifically to more than one cell type. In the case of C3/1 the specific binding in adult skeletal muscle is not only to satellite cells but also to peripheral nerve Schwann cells (Fig. 17). Satellite and Schwann cells are derived from different layers of the early embryo, and there was no *a priori* reason to imagine a common molecular entity shared by these two cell types but not by others (see section 5).

Figure 13. Phase contrast micrographs of 5-day-old muscle culture 24 hr after treatment with hybridoma antibody #6. Postfusion myogenic cell cultures were treated with 1 μg/ ml purified antibody with 5% guinea pig complement in complete medium at 37°C for 2 hr. After this period, during which most mononucleated cells had lysed and retracted off the dish, the cultures were rinsed and returned to the incubator for 24 hr. Such procedures routinely result in myogenic cultures in which 97% of viable nuclei were in multinucleated cells.

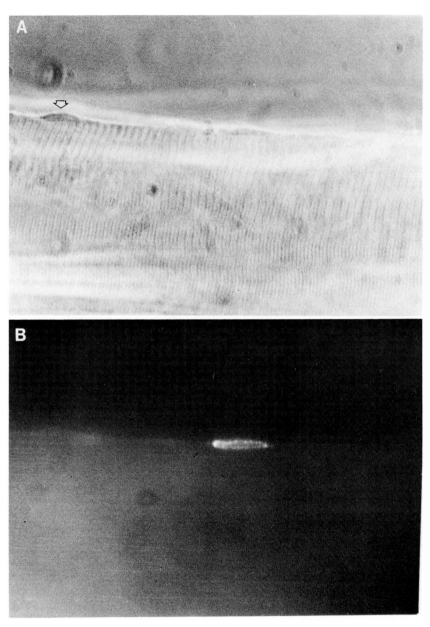

Figure 15. Phase micrograph (A) and fluorescence micrograph (B) of teased adult chicken muscle fiber after staining with FITC-labeled monoclonal antibody C3/1. Note selective staining of satellite cell. Structure at arrow in (A) is probably a fibroblast.

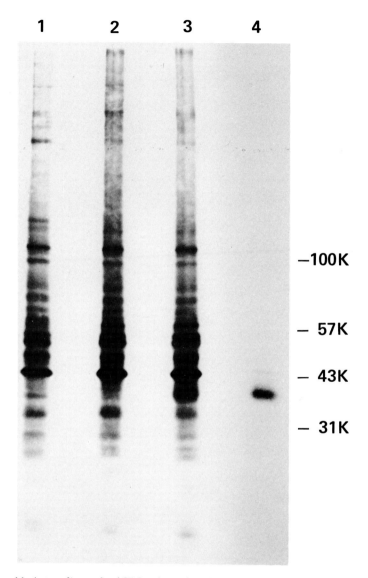

Figure 16. Autoradiograph of SDS-polyacrylamide gel (5–15% gradient) after electrophoresis of ^{35}S-labeled samples. Samples were prepared from a 1% Triton X-100 extract of chick myoblasts after overnight labeling with [^{35}S]methionine. Samples were: lane 1: unfractionated lysate; lane 2; lysate material nonspecifically binding to Sepharose beads coupled with MOPC-21 IgG; lane 3: lysate material binding to Sepharose beads coupled with monoclonal antibody C3/1; lane 4: lysate material eluted from C3/1 Sepharose beads with 0.1 M triethylamine and affinity purified by a second cycle through C3/1 Sepharose beads. Radioisotope content of the samples was adjusted to give resolvable electrophoretic bands upon autoradiography. Calculations indicate that the polypeptide specifically binding C3/1 Sepharose may contain about 0.0005 of total radiation in the lysate.

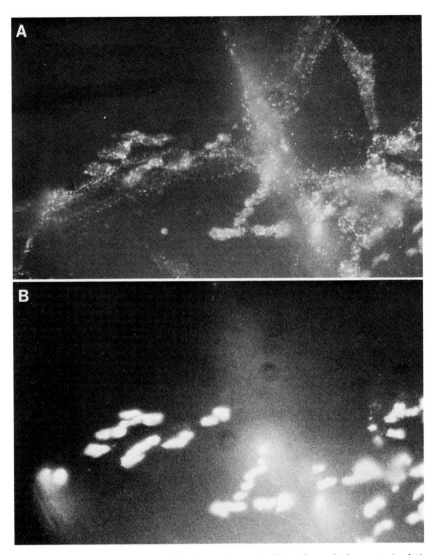

Figure 17. Fluorescence micrographs of teased muscle fibers from chicken anterior latissimus dorsi muscle. The same field is shown in (A) stained with C3/1 antibody and fluorescein-labeled rabbit anti-mouse IgG, and in (B) stained with tetraethylrhodamine-labeled α-bungarotoxin. Schwann cells over nerve terminals and axons show stippled fluorescence in A.

4.3. Monoclonal Antibodies to Extracellular Matrix Proteins

Another aspect of muscle biology receiving increasing attention in our laboratory is analysis of the extracellular connective tissue components which surround skeletal muscle fibers. Here, too, monoclonal antibodies provide specific and sensitive probes for identification and characterization of the molecules of interest. The importance of extracellular matrix with respect to the organization of the supporting groundwork of tissue, to the shaping of organs, and to the control of morphogenetic movements has long been recognized. More recently it has become clear that highly specific cell surface properties may involve molecular species present in the zone extending away from the plasma membrane. In muscle this acellular exoskeletal sheath includes the basal lamina, closely apposed to the cell membrane, and extends into a variety of complicated and still uncharacterized three-dimensional structures and networks with increasing distance from the cell. The collagens, elastin, laminin, proteoglycans, fibronectin, and hyaluronic acid (along with some as yet ill-defined glycoproteins) are probably primary constituents of extracellular matrices.

4.3.1. Analysis of Fibronectin Biosynthesis, Secretion, and Organization.
The current view that the matrix is the product of connective tissue cells (e.g., fibroblasts, chondrocytes, and osteocytes) is undergoing revision. This has resulted from the findings that some matrix components are also synthesized by nonconnective tissue cells (Kurkinen and Alitalo, 1979; Alitalo et al., 1980). Of particular interest in this regard is fibronectin, which has been reported to be distributed on the sarcolemma of adult striated muscle (Stenman and Vaheri, 1978; Krieg et al., 1979). Furthermore, reports have appeared of changes in fibronectin distribution and accumulation during the differentiation of myoblasts to myotubes in clonal muscle cell lines in vitro (Hynes et al., 1976; Chen, 1977; Furcht et al., 1978). We have carried out similar studies of fibronectin biosynthesis secretion and extracellular organization during myogenesis in vitro, but have used primary cultures of embryonic muscle cells and monoclonal antibody techniques. The results have interested implications for muscle cell surface differentiation, as well as the production and organization of matrix components by muscle cells. This study also illustrates a variety of techniques which will be important in designing similar studies concerning other components of extracellular matrix.

A monoclonal antibody to fibronectin was generated from hybridization of Sp 2/0 myeloma nonsecretor cells with spleen cells of a mouse which had been immunized with chick embryo fibroblast fibronectin. The antigen had been purified by differential extraction and chromatography on an affinity column of collagen. The initial screening for positive hybridoma clones involved antibody binding assays to live muscle cultures, using iodinated or fluoresceinated second antibody specific for mouse immunoglobulin. Cloning in soft agar and further assays led to the selection of a single IgG-producing clone. The IgG produced by this clone bound to and, in the presence of goat anti-mouse IgG antibody, precipitated (1) cell-surface-derived fibronectin, (2) secreted fibronectin, and (3) secreted cold-insoluble globulin (a circulatory form of fibronectin). The antibody proved to be specific for chick fibronectin and did not react with fibronectins from horse serum or calf serum. This factor has had important experimental consequences, for it has allowed analysis of the production and distribution of endogenous fibronectin in both chick muscle and fibroblast cultures, even though exogenous fibronectin was present in the serum component of the culture medium. (Our chick embryo extract does not contain a detectable quantity of fibronectin.) Figure 18 illustrates the selective immunoprecipitation of [^{35}S]methionine-labeled fibronectin from culture medium containing metabolically labeled muscle secretory proteins. The principle labeled secretory component in the immunoprecipitate is the fibronectin 230,000-dalton component, which is quantitatively precipitated under these conditions.

Because both fibroblasts and myogenic cells synthesize fibronectin, the "deep six" cytotoxicity treatment (see above) was necessary in order to generate essentially "pure" myotube cultures. Such cultures could be used to examine the kinetics of biosynthesis and secretion of fibronectin. Figure 19 illustrates the appearance of labeled secretory fibronectin in the culture medium as a function of time after the introduction of [^{35}S]methionine. Secretion of soluble fibronectin can be detected about 2–3 hr after addition of label. During a chase with unlabeled methionine, or following inhibition of protein synthesis, fibronectin secretion continues for about 2 hr. In these aspects the kinetics of fibronectin production resemble those described for AChE biosynthesis and secretion. In fact, analysis of the labeled secretory proteins of "pure" skeletal muscle cultures by SDS gel electrophoresis suggests that similar kinetics of synthesis and secretion pertain to all of the major secretory proteins.

Fibronectin biosynthesis and secretion have also been studied in chick embryo fibroblasts. In these cells, which should be metabolically similar to the fibroblasts present in ordinary primary muscle cultures, the intracellular transport time is only about 30 min (as opposed to 2–3 hours for myotubes) (Fig. 19). Furthermore, these fibroblasts appear to make and secrete fibronectin at a rate about five times greater per nucleus than do myotubes. Thus, it was imperative to remove fibroblast

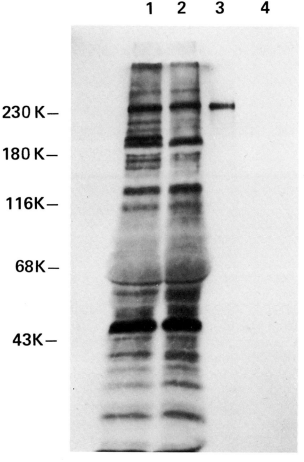

Figure 18. Analysis of [^{35}S]methionine-labeled secretory proteins of chick myotube cultures. Purified myotube cultures were labeled overnight with [^{35}S]methionine, and the secretory proteins present in the conditioned medium were analyzed by SDS PAGE (5–15% gradient gel) followed by autoradiography (lane 1). An equal aliquot of labeled conditioned medium was digested with 20 units of purified bacterial collagenased (Advanced Biofactures) for 60 min at 37°C and electrophoresed (lane 2). Note the loss of several high-molecular bands indicating that muscle cells are synthesizing several forms of procollagen peptides. Incubation of conditioned medium with monoclonal antifibronectin antibody followed by rabbit anti-mouse IgG second antibody resulted in precipitation of secreted fibronectins (lane 3). No precipitated labeled proteins were observed when MOPC-21 IgG was used as the first antibody (lane 4).

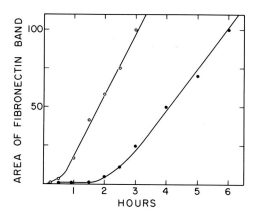

Figure 19. Kinetics of secretion of [^{35}S]methionine-labeled fibronectin into the culture medium during continuous labeling of chick myotube cultures (●—●—●—●) or tertiary chick embryo fibroblast cultures (○—○—○—○) with [^{35}S]methionine. Note lag before acceleration of secretion rate to steady level. The time lag is relatively brief for fibroblast fibronectin secretion (30 min) compared with that observed for pure myotube cultures (2–3 hr). Analysis of fibronectin secretion involved immunoprecipitation of secreted fibronectin with monoclonal antifibronectin antibody and second antibody (Fig. 18) and quantification of radiation after electrophoresis of immunoprecipitates on SDS polyacrylamide gels.

contamination in order to reliably measure myotube fibronectin secretion.

An interesting outcome of this study was that only about 15% of secretory fibronectin is actually released in soluble form from the myotubes. The remaining 85% of the fibronectin synthesized in these muscle cultures remains bound to either the cells or the culture dish. This fibronectin is trypsin sensitive, and its accumulation can therefore be measured during labeling with [^{35}S]methionine. As in the case of integral membrane proteins described above, fibronectin begins to appear at the cell surface between 2 and 3 hr after the beginning of the labeling period. Thereafter its accumulation is approximately linear with time.

The accumulation of total cell- and dish-bound fibronectin has been studied as a function of time in cell culture, with the aid of our monoclonal chick-specific antifibronectin antibody directly labeled with rhodamine or fluorescein (Fig. 20). These experiments reveal that there is a slow build-up of fibronectin associated with the collagenous substratum of the culture dish. An intensely staining fibrillar matrix is often associated with solitary myoblasts, especially at the ends of the bipolar cells where attachment to the substratum occurs. As the myogenic cells align prior to fusion, this matrix becomes more prominent, and immediately prior to fusion, punctate accumulations of fibronectin occur at sites of cell contact. Little fibronectin is associated with the surface of newly formed myotubes. As they mature, however, deposits of fibronectin accumulate under the myotubes and fibrils containing fibronectin extend over their upper surface.

An additional observation of interest is that intracellular pools of newly synthesized fibronectin can be visualized after immunofluorescent labeling of permeabilized fibroblasts or myotubes. These pools appear to be localized within perinuclear granules, consistent with the possibility that the major fraction of intracellular fibronectin is localized with the intracellular pool of newly synthesized AChRs, in the Golgi apparatus.

4.3.2. *Other Extracellular Matrix Antigens.* Not only are myotubes capable of secreting fibronectin, but they also secrete a variety of other polypeptides. This is illustrated in Fig. 18. Presumably many of these products, like fibronectin, are destined for incorporation into extracellular matrix. Monoclonal antibodies provide a means by which to identify different extracellular matrix components *in vivo*. These same components can then be traced *in vitro*. Figure 21 illustrates staining patterns obtained with different monoclonal antibodies on frozen sectioned chicken skeletal muscle. Even at the light-microscopic level differences in antigen distribution and substructure are apparent. Such differences suggest that our antibodies recognize a variety of matrix constituents and demonstrate the complex organization of muscle extracellular matrix *in vivo*. Further, when the same antibodies are used to stain embryonic chick muscle cultures it becomes clear not only that these antigens accumulate *in vitro* but that they become assembled into an orderly structure. These observations indicate the cultures elaborate an *in vitro* approximation of the extracellular matrix found *in vivo*.

Culture provides the opportunity to analyze the relation between soluble proteins secreted by various cell types and insoluble matrix components. The antibodies used to define antigen distribution can also be used to identify the antigens biochemically. Our findings using antibody #39 illustrate this point. The distribution of #39 antigen *in vivo* is shown in Fig. 21. The antigen is present both in the endomysium around individual muscle fibers and in the perimysium which surrounds bundles of fibers. The staining of perimysium indicates that the antigen is a component of reticular connective tissue, and while possibly the antigen might extend into the basal lamina, it is certainly not limited to that region. In culture, discrete patches of #39 matrix accumulate on the surfaces of myotubes. We find that some of these patches coincide with AChR clusters on the myotubes (see below).

Using antibody #39 we have been able to identify soluble antigen among the secreted products synthesized in primary chicken muscle cultures (containing myotubes and fibroblasts). Figure 22 shows the

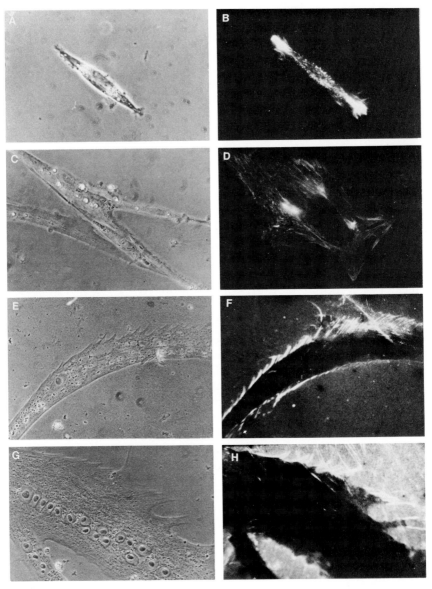

Figure 20. Double immunofluorescent localization of fibronectin during myogenesis. (A, B) Phase and fluorescent views of a solitary myoblast 24 hr after plating, stained by indirect immunofluorescence with monoclonal antifibronectin antibody followed by fluorescein-tagged goat anti-mouse antibody. Forty-eight hours after plating, myogenic cells in the process of aligning and fusing are surrounded by fibrillar network of fibronectin with dense accumulations at sites of close cell–cell contact (C, D). In well-developed postfusion myotube cultures (6 days after plating) deposits of fibronectin accumulate under the cells,

results of a double-antibody precipitation from culture medium containing [^{35}S]methionine-labeled secreted products. Antibody #39 specifically precipitates a doublet of bands with molecular masses of approximately 130,000 and 140,000 daltons as well as a polypeptide with an apparent molecular mass of about 255,000 daltons. Biochemical characterization of these peptides is now underway. We are also examining the cellular origin of #39 antigen and are interested in determining the relation of this antigen to other matrix components during matrix biogenesis.

4.3.3. *Basal Lamina Antigens.* The interaction of extracellular matrix and plasmalemma is currently a topic of much interest. Among the various extracellular matrix antigens defined by our library of monoclonal antibodies one group may be especially relevant. These antibodies appear to recognize components situated within the basal lamina, that region of the extracellular matrix immediately adjacent to the plasma membrane. The basal lamina of skeletal muscle is not well characterized. Chemically it is known to contain both collagenous and noncollagenous proteins. Morphologically it is organized into a meshwork of fine fibrils on the outer surface of the plasmalemma, and it is the only component of the extracellular matrix to enter the synaptic cleft at the neuromuscular junction (see, for example, Heuser and Salpeter, 1979). Within the synaptic cleft the basal lamina appears to be chemically specialized in that it contains a high concentration of the junctional AChE (Hall, 1973; McMahan *et al.*, 1978). Recent studies further suggest that the basal lamina at neuromuscular junctions may contain chemical specializations capable of inducing the development of both "synaptic" vesicles and "junctional" AChR aggregates in regenerating amphibian nerve and muscle cells, respectively (Sanes *et al.*, 1978; Burden *et al.*, 1979).

As defined by several monoclonal antibodies we have prepared both against chick and frog tissues, basal lamina antigens show a number of features which can readily be distinguished by immunocytochemical techniques at the level of the light microscope. On adult muscle fibers, for example, they are distributed over the entire cell surface and, unlike the other extracellular markers, extend into the synaptic cleft of the neuromuscular junction. Some of them are also associated with blood vessels, including capillaries. The localization of basal lamina antigens at the neuromuscular junction can most directly be demonstrated by

---

and fibrils containing fibronectin extend from the upper cell surface and the edge of the cells to points of substrate contact away from the myotubes (E, F). Ten days after plating, dense fibronectin fibrils remain associated with the myotube cell surface (G, H). Also note the accumulation of a uniform mat of fibronectin bound to the collagenous substratum of the cultures.

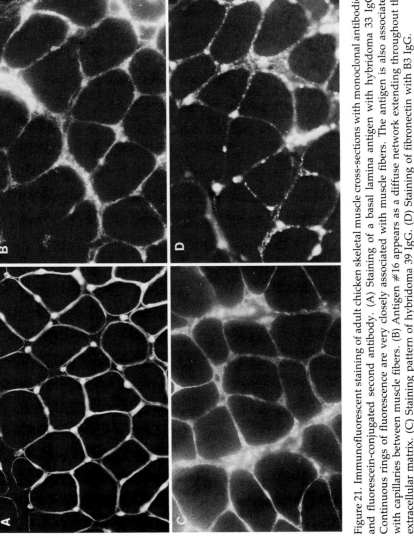

Figure 21. Immunofluorescent staining of adult chicken skeletal muscle cross-sections with monoclonal antibodies and fluorescein-conjugated second antibody. (A) Staining of a basal lamina antigen with hybridoma 33 IgG. Continuous rings of fluorescence are very closely associated with muscle fibers. The antigen is also associated with capillaries between muscle fibers. (B) Antigen #16 appears as a diffuse network extending throughout the extracellular matrix. (C) Staining pattern of hybridoma 39 IgG. (D) Staining of fibronectin with B3 IgG.

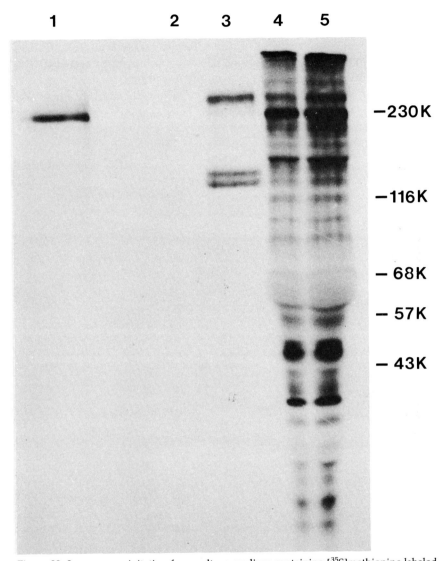

Figure 22. Immunoprecipitation from culture medium containing [³⁵S]methionine labeled secreted products. Conventional (fibroblast-containing) muscle cultures were labeled with [³⁵S]methionine for 24 hr and the conditioned medium used for double-antibody precipitations. Products were separated on 5–15% gradient SDS polyacrylamide gels and analyzed by autoradiography. Lane 1: precipitation of fibronectin with monoclonal antibody B3. Lane 2: control with MOPC 21 IgG from the P3 × 63 myeloma line. Lane 3: selective precipitation of #39 antigen. Lanes 4 and 5: profiles of [³⁵S]methionine-labeled secreted products.

comparing their distribution with that of α-bungarotoxin which binds to junctional accumulations of AChRs. Some basal lamina antigens show substantial concentration at neuromuscular junctions (Fig. 23).

While such local chemical specialization is not unexpected at the adult neuromuscular junction, one might not anticipate a similar level of structural complexity on embryonic muscle cells developing in the

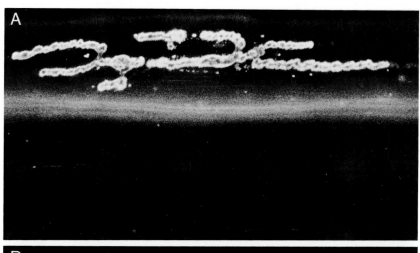

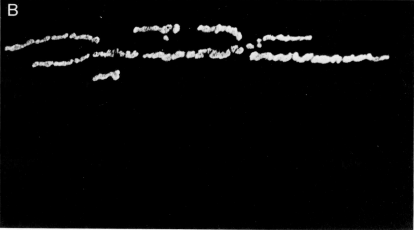

Figure 23. Localization of basal lamina antigens at the adult frog neuromuscular junction. Fluorescence micrographs of isolated *Xenopus* muscle fibers stained (A) with monoclonal antibody followed by fluorescein-labeled goat anti-mouse IgG, or (B) with tetramethyl-rhodamine-labeled α-bungarotoxin to visualize postjunctional AChRs. Note the corresponding distributions of the two markers, and a diffuse labeling of the entire muscle fiber with antibody.

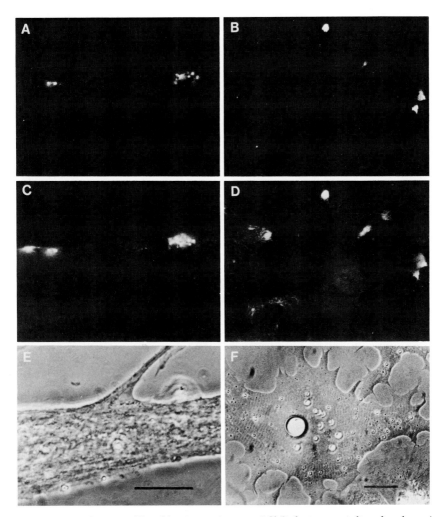

Figure 24. Localization of basal lamina antigens at AChR clusters on cultured embryonic muscle cells. Phase contrast and fluorescence micrographs of chick and frog muscle cells in culture. (A, B) Chick and *Xenopus* muscle cells, respectively, stained with tetramethyl-rhodamine-labeled α-bungarotoxin, which reveals discrete clusters of densely packed AChRs in the sarcolemma. (C, D) Same fields as (A, B), stained with fluorescein-labeled antibody toward local accumulations of basal lamina antigens over each of the receptor clusters. (E, F) Phase contrast views of the fields shown above. The bar in (E) represents 30 μm in (A, C, and E); the bar in (F) represents 30 μm in (B, D, and F).

isolation of a tissue culture dish. Surprisingly, however, similar immunocytochemical experiments in embryonic muscle cells from both the chick and the frog reveal that a variety of specializations of basal lamina antigens are on the cell surface and that some of these contain localized high concentrations of AChRs (Fig. 24). Although we observe antigen patches not associated with AChR clusters, we never observe receptor clusters without associated antigen. Apparently, even in the absence of innervation muscle cells have the capacity to generate extensive regional specializations of their surface analogous to that at the neuromuscular junction. Direct links between plasma membrane and extracellular matrix organization are strongly supported by this coordination of distribution, which extends to a striking congruence in shape between the AChR cluster and its overlying patch of basal lamina. Taken together with their time course of appearance, where basal lamina patches seem to precede AChR clusters, organization of the basal lamina may possibly play a directive role in determining the surface organization of AChRs within the sarcolemma.

Antigen #39 also shows a somewhat patchy distribution on cultured myotubes, and some of these patches coincide with AChE clusters on the myotubes. While the correspondence in distribution of AChRs and #39 antigen in such regions is striking, the relation between antigen and receptor appears to be complex. Only some AChR clusters have associated antigen while others lack any detectable staining. Furthermore, the distribution of antigen *in vivo* suggests that #39 may not be present in substantial amounts within the basal lamina. It thus would seem reasonable to predict that any interaction between AChRs and this antigen is likely to be an indirect one. One interpretation of these observations is that the basal lamina plays a role both in AChR organization and in the build-up of more distal extracellular structures.

5. DISCUSSION

Monoclonal antibodies have provided a means to investigate problems related to the cell biology and biochemistry of muscle surface structures. Most obviously, monoclonal antibodies represent specific, often high-affinity ligands for molecules of interest. Further, the production of such antibodies does not require purification of an identified antigen or even prior knowledge of its existence. Most of our useful monoclonal antibodies derive from immunizations with complex, poorly characterized mixtures of antigens. Immunocytochemical techniques, employing ^{125}I- or fluorescent-labeled second antibody, provide rapid assessment of the cellular location of antigen—surface vs. internal (Fig. 10), muscle fiber vs. fibroblast vs. myoblast (Fig. 13)—and provide semiquantitative information concerning relative antigen density on different cells (Fig. 13). Since substantial quantities of individual purified monoclonal antibodies can be generated with relatively modest effort, material is available for antibody-consumptive uses such as production of affinity adsorbants for antigen purification (Fig. 16).

Although the value of monoclonal antibodies in neurobiological research is hardly in doubt, they often present unexpected technical difficulties. Despite superficial similarities to conventional immunochemical reagents, monoclonal antibodies are often quite unlike antisera. While normal antisera have properties of a diverse molecular population of ligands, a monoclonal antibody has the unique properties of a single molecular species of immunoglobulin. On the one hand, this purity allows one to avoid the single overwhelming qualification inherent in use of conventional antisera, that is, questionable chemical specificity. Often it is impossible to rigorously demonstrate that an antiserum interacts only with a single molecular species. Immunochemical specificity is, indeed, often *less* than the purity of the macromolecule used as antigen. On the other hand, the uniqueness of each monoclonal antibody results in different problems, in both technique and interpretation.

In the course of our work we have encountered several kinds of technical problems. First, individual monoclonal antibodies may be exquisitely sensitive to derivatization. For example, our antibody #24 is completely inactivated by chloramine-T-catalyzed iodination; antibody #33 is greatly impaired by derivatization of ϵ-amino groups (as in fluorescein conjugation). Likewise, because monoclonal antibodies recognize single determinants on their target antigens, the antigenic sites may themselves be quite sensitive to chemical modification. Thus, glutaraldehyde fixation eliminates roughly half of the antigens defined by our first 20 monoclonal antibodies, and formaldehyde fixation greatly damages about one-fourth. Other antigens are destroyed by reduction or denaturation. Second, immunocytochemical selection procedures such as fluorescent double-antibody staining (Figs. 10 and 21) do not necessarily eliminate weakly binding antibodies. We have in fact observed a wide range of affinities and avidities among selected monoclonal antibodies for their antigens. In one case we have examined carefully, there is a very strong temperature dependence in dissociation rate, the antigen–antibody complex appearing stable at 0°C but dissociating with a half-time of about 10 min at 37°C. Third, as mentioned above, many monoclonal antibodies are nonprecipitating, presumably due to a low valency of the antigenic groups on the target macromolecule. Fourth, because of isotypic purity of monoclonal antibodies, some classical immunological techniques, such as *Staphylococcus* protein A binding and complement fixation, may not be applicable. A large number of our monoclonal antibodies are IgGl, which do not bind protein A or fix complement. Isotypic purity also complicates the design of controls, such as testing for nonspecific binding. In our experience, IgMs have a much higher level of nonspecific binding, so that in some screening assays nonspecifically bound IgM gives a false positive signal compared with an IgG control.

We are also aware of several problems of interpretation of results obtained with monoclonal antibodies. One is related to the point made immediately above. Since each monoclonal antibody is a unique macromolecule, there is no perfect negative control to use, for example, in binding and in immunoprecipitation experiments. In addition, we have encountered a number of examples of cross-reactivity of monoclonal antibodies with two or more cell types. For example, antibody C3/1, which appears to bind to a 38,000-dalton peptide of myoblast and myotube plasma membranes, also binds to a determinant on Schwann cells (Fig. 17). This surprising result might indicate a common molecule in the membranes of the two cell types. Perhaps a less likely but intriguing possibility is that the result could be due to a pair of quite different molecules sharing a common antigenic determinant. The odds against such a coincidence may not be so great as generally imagined. There is increasing evidence that evolution has proceeded in part by gene duplication and then sequence divergence. Thus, sequence homologies between heretofore seemingly unrelated proteins are being discovered. We foresee the possibility that many mistaken "identities" will be announced in the coming years, perhaps, for example, when monoclonal antibodies are used as a means of defining cell populations in the nervous system.

Monoclonal antibody technology has led us in new directions. We observed components of the extracellular matrix appearing during myogenesis and were led to ask about the complexity, organization, and sources of the material. We observed developmentally regulated antigens which come and go on different schedules and have probed further into the complexity of developmental expression in myogenesis. We discovered an antigen which might facilitate identification and further study of satellite cells in adult muscle and have been led to characterize it. We came upon a method for generating virtually pure myotube cultures and thus could go on to explore fibronectin biogenesis and its secretion from myotubes and to explore the other secretory capacities of these cells. We have gained greater appreciation of the muscle fiber surface as an intricate multilayered structure within which many specific associative interactions must occur. There must be, in a sense, "receptors" within the plasma membrane for some of the extracellular matrix elements of the basal lamina. Likewise we must expect to find further specific interactions between basal lamina components and more peripheral elements of extracellular matrix. Several newly discovered antigens should facilitate analysis of turnover rates of integral membrane proteins. The monoclonal antibodies against surface and secretory components will allow further studies on the possibility of coupled secretion and membrane biogenesis. The monoclonal antibodies to extracellular matrix antigens that co-localize with AChR clusters on cultured *Xenopus* and chick muscle and are concentrated at neuromuscular junctions provide a means for examining specific matrix–plasma membrane interactions and forces which may be involved in synaptogenesis.

ACKNOWLEDGMENTS

Research in the authors' laboratory is supported in part by grants from the Muscular Dystrophy Association and the National Institutes of Health. We wish to thank Mrs. Delores Somerville for technical assistance.

6. REFERENCES

Alitalo, K., Kurkinen, M., Vaheri, A., Virtanen, I., Rohde, H., and Timpl, R., 1980, Basal lamina glycoproteins are produced by neuroblastoma cells, *Nature (London)* **287:**465.
Appel, S. H., Anwyl, R., McAdams, M. W., and Elias, S., 1977, Accelerated degradation of acetylcholine receptor from cultured rat myotubes with myasthenia gravis sera and globulins, *Proc. Natl. Acad. Sci. U.S.A.* **74:**2130.
Berg, D. K., and Hall, Z. W., 1975, Loss of α-bungarotoxin from junctional and extrajunctional acetylcholine receptors in rat diaphragm *in vivo* and in organ culture, *J. Physiol. (London)* **252:**771.
Burden, S., 1977, Development of the neuromuscular junction in the chick embryo: The number, distribution, and stability of acetylcholine receptors, *Dev. Biol.* **57:**317.
Burden, S. J., Sargent, P. B., and McMahan, U. J., 1979, Acetylcholine receptors in regenerating muscle accumulate at original sites in the absence of the nerve, *J. Cell Biol.* **82:**412.
Chang, C. C., and Huang, M. C., 1975, Turnover of junctional and extrajunctional acetylcholine receptors of rat diaphragm, *Nature (London)* **253:**643.
Chen, L., 1977, Alteration in cell surface LETS protein during myogenesis, *Cell* **10:**393.
Devreotes, P. N., and Fambrough, D. M., 1976a, Synthesis of the acetylcholine receptor by cultured chick myotubes and denervated mouse extensor digitorum longus muscles, *Proc. Natl. Acad. Sci. U.S.A.* **73:**161.

Devreotes, P. N., and Fambrough, D. M., 1976b, Turnover of acetylcholine receptors in skeletal muscle, *Cold Spring Harbor Symp. Quant. Biol.* **40**:237.

Devreotes, P. N., Gardner, J. M., and Fambrough, D. M., 1977, Kinetics of biosynthesis of acetylcholine receptor and subsequent incorporation into plasma membrane of cultured chick skeletal muscle, *Cell* **10**:365.

Fambrough, D. M., 1979, Control of acetylcholine receptors in skeletal muscle, *Physiol. Rev.* **59**:165.

Fambrough, D. M., and Devreotes, P. N., 1978, Newly synthesized acetylcholine receptors are located in the Golgi apparatus, *J. Cell Biol.* **76**:237.

Fambrough, D. M. and Rash, J. E., 1971, Development of acetylcholine sensitivity during myogenesis, *Dev. Biol.* **26**:55.

Fambrough, D. M., Drachman, D. B., and Satyamurti, S., 1973, Neuromuscular junction in myasthenia gravis: Decreased acetylcholine receptors, *Science* **182**:293.

Fambrough, D. M., Devreotes, P. N., Card, D. J., Gardner, J., and Tepperman, K., 1978, Metabolism of acetylcholine receptors in skeletal muscle, *Natl. Cancer Inst.* **48**:277.

Furcht, L. T., Mosher, D. F., and Wendelschafer-Crabb, G., 1978, Immunocytochemical localization of fibronectin (LETS protein) on the surface of L6 myoblasts: Light and electron microscope studies, *Cell* **13**:263.

Galfre, G., Howe, S. C., Milstein, C., Butcher, G. W., and Howard, J. C., 1977, Antibodies to major histocompatibility antigens produced by hybrid cell lines, *Nature (London)* **266**:550.

Gardner, J. M., and Fambrough, D. M., 1979, Acetylcholine receptor degradation measured by density labeling: Effects of cholinergic ligands and evidence against recycling, *Cell* **16**:661.

Hall, Z. W., 1973, Multiple forms of acetylcholinesterase and their distribution in endplate and non-endplate regions of rat diaphragm muscle, *J. Neurobiol.* **4**:343.

Hartzell, H. C., and Fambrough, D. M., 1973, Acetylcholine receptor production and incorporation into membranes of developing muscle fibers, *Dev. Biol.* **30**:153.

Heinemann, S., Bevan, S., Kullberg, R., Lindstrom, J., and Rice, J., 1977, Modulation of acetylcholine receptor by antibody against the receptor, *Proc. Natl. Acad. Sci. U.S.A.* **74**:3090.

Heuser, J. E. and Salpeter, S. R., 1979, Organization of acetylcholine receptors in quick-frozen, deep-etched, and rotary-replicated *Torpedo* postsynaptic membrane, *J. Cell Biol.* **82**:150.

Hynes, R. O., Martin, G. S., Shearer, M., Critchley, D. R., and Epstein, G. J., 1976, Viral transformation of rat myoblasts: Effects on fusion and surface properties, *Dev. Biol.* **48**:35.

Kao, I., and Drachman, D. B., 1977, Myasthenic immunoglobulin accelerates acetylcholine receptor degradation, *Science* **196**:527.

Kennett, R. H., Denis, K. A., Tung, A. S., and Klinman, N. R., 1978, Hybrid plasmacytoma production: Fusions with adult spleen cells, monoclonal spleen fragments, neonatal spleen cells and human spleen cells, *Curr. Top. Microbiol. Immunol.* **81**:77.

Kohler, G., and Milstein, C., 1975, Continuous cultures of fused cells secreting antibody of predefined specificity, *Nature (London)* **256**:495.

Krieg, T., Timpl, R., Alitalo, K., Kurkinen, M., and Vaheri, A., 1979, Type III procollagen is the major collagenous component produced by a continuous rhabdomyosarcoma cell line, *FEBS Lett.* **104**:405.

Kurkinen, M., and Alitalo, K., 1979, Fibronectin and procollagen produced by a clonal line of Schwann cells, *FEBS Lett.* **102**:64.

Linden, D. C., and Fambrough, D. M., 1979, Biosynthesis and degradation of acetylcholine receptors in rat skeletal muscles. Effects of electrical stimulation, *Neuroscience* **4**:527.

Lomo, T., and Westgaard, R. H., 1975, Further studies on the control of ACh sensitivity by muscle activity in the rat, *J. Physiol. (London)* **252**:603.

Loring, R., and Salpeter, M. M., 1980, Denervation increases turnover of junctional acetylcholine receptors, *Proc. Natl. Acad. Sci. U.S.A.* **77**:2293.

Massoulie, J., Bon, S., and Vigny, M., 1980, The polymorphism of cholinesterases in vertebrates, *Neurochem. Int.* **2**:161.

McMahan, U. J., Sanes, J. R., and Marshall, L. M., 1978, Cholinesterase is associated with the basal lamina at the neuromuscular junction, *Nature (London)* **271**:172.

Noble, M. D., Brown, T. H., and Peacock, J. H., 1978, Regulation of acetylcholine receptor levels by a cholinergic agonist in mouse muscle cell cultures, *Proc. Natl. Acad. Sci. U.S.A.* **75**:3488.

Reiness, C. G., and Hall, Z. W., 1977, Electrical stimulation of denervated muscles reduces incorporation of methionine into the ACh receptor, *Nature (London)* **268**:655.

Rotundo, R. L., and Fambrough, D. M., 1980a, Synthesis, transport and fate of acetylcholinesterase in cultured chick embryo muscle cells, *Cell* **22**:583.

Rotundo, R. L., and Fambrough, D. M., 1980b, Secretion of acetylcholinesterase: Relation to acetylcholine receptor metabolism, *Cell* **22**:595.

Rotundo, R. L., Gardner, J. M., Bayne, E. K., Wakshull, E., Anderson, M. J., and Fambrough, D. M., 1980, Cell surface and secretory glycoproteins of skeletal muscle, *Carnegie Inst. Washington Yearb.* **79**:19.

Sanes, J. R., Marshall, L. M., and McMahan, U. J., 1978, Reinnervation of muscle fiber basal lamina after removal of myofibers: Differentiation of regenerating axons at original synaptic sites, *J. Cell Biol.* **78**:176.

Stenman, S., and Vaheri, A., 1978, Distribution of a major connective tissue protein, fibronectin, in normal human tissues, *J. Exp. Med.* **147**:1054.

3

Monoclonal Antibodies to Synaptic Constituents

WILLIAM D. MATTHEW, ERIC OUTWATER,
LARISA TSAVALER, and LOUIS F. REICHARDT

1. INTRODUCTION

The major goal of our laboratory is to understand how chemical synapses are formed, maintained, and modified during development. We are trying to delineate the sequence of events that occurs during synapse formation and identify the molecular changes that underlie this sequence of interaction between defined neuronal and target types.

A prerequisite for this work is a more detailed knowledge of the molecular composition of the synapse. Extensive efforts, most notably by Mahler, Cotman, Matus, Siekevitz and collaborators, have been directed to the purification of synaptic junctions (cf. Mahler, 1977; Matus and Taff-Jones, 1978). As discussed by these investigators, even the best preparations are likely to be heavily contaminated with nonsynaptic and even nonneuronal material. Adequate assays for purification are not available, particularly for distinguishing synaptic and nonsynaptic neuronal membrane. All these preparations contain synaptic material from a variety of cell types, and recently it has become clear that synaptic preparations from different brain regions contain different spectra of

WILLIAM D. MATTHEW, ERIC OUTWATER, LARISA TSAVALER, and LOUIS F. REICHARDT · Department of Physiology, University of California, San Francisco, Calif. 94143.

proteins (Carlin *et al.*, 1980). The only absolutely convincing localization studies have used immunohistochemical criteria (Wood *et al.*, 1980; Bloom *et al.*, 1979; Matus and Taff-Jones, 1978).

Immunological probes, recognizing particular types of neurons, synapses, or other structures, have great potential for identifying cell classes and lineages, purifying cells or organelles on principles independent of classical physical methods, and monitoring changes during development. Antisera now exist that define the major cell types of the nervous system (cf. Raff *et al.*, 1979). Antibodies against transmitter enzymes and transmitter substances have provided internal markers to distinguish subclasses of neurons (cf. Wood *et al.*, 1976; Stell *et al.*, 1980; Hokfelt *et al.*, 1980), revealing a diversity of cell type and function that had been suspected, but not clearly established previously. Since monoclonal antibodies recognize single antigenic determinants in a complex immunogen, they circumvent many of the problems neurobiologists face in raising specific antisera when equipped with the impure populations of cells or organelles currently available. In this report, we will demonstrate that monoclonal antibodies raised against rat brain synaptic junctions show great specificity for different cell types and organelles, and will illustrate the use of these sera in purifications and developmental studies.

2. PREPARATION OF SYNAPTIC JUNCTIONS AND HYBRIDOMA ANTIBODIES

We have prepared several hundred cell lines secreting monoclonal antibodies against synaptic membrane constituents from rat brain and *Torpedo* electroplax synaptosomes. Preparations of synaptic membranes, junctional complexes, and postsynaptic densities were prepared with standard physical separations based on size, density, and detergent resistance (cf. Matus and Taff-Jones, 1978). In the antibodies raised against rat brain preparations, we anticipated detecting antigens that were shared by many different classes of synapses in addition to neuronal surface antigens and antigens localized to contaminating membranes from other cell types. The *Torpedo* electroplax provides the best currently available source for one class of nerve terminal—in this case a cholinergic synapse very closely related to the neuromuscular junction. From these immunizations, we have anticipated defining antigens with more restricted distributions in the nervous system that will be useful in studying cholinergic development and synapse formation. The hybridomas derived from *Torpedo* were prepared by Dr. P. Kushner in this laboratory, but will not be discussed in this report.

In our initial experiments, the spleen cells from immunized mice were fused to the NS-1 nonsecreting myeloma cell line, and the mixture was then plated at a clonal dilution in selective media. After hybrid cells had grown up in culture, a standard solid-phase radioimmune assay was used to screen the hybridoma antibodies (Klinman, 1972). Antisera that bound synaptic membranes were screened against kidney, liver, spleen, and thymus membrane preparations. Only the clones whose antibodies appeared to be brain specific were maintained. The vast majority, however, of our monoclonal antibodies to molecules enriched in synapses have been isolated using an immunohistochemical screen on frozen sections of retina or cerebellum, tissues where antibodies that bind to synaptic regions are easily recognized. Roughly 5% of the initial hybridoma lines have appeared promising by this test. Single cells have been isolated in micropipets and used to generate unambiguously clonal lines for further study. Some of the antibodies secreted by these cell lines define antigens present in such low concentrations that they would not have been recognized in solid-phase assays.

Some general properties of the antigens defined by a selective sample of these antisera are summarized in Table I. A small number of hybridoma cell lines have been characterized that distinguish the major cell types found in cultures of neuronal material. Representatives, illustrated in Fig. 1, bind the surface of neurons, the surface of oligodendrocytes, or the intermediate filaments of astrocytes and fibroblasts. The antibodies to the surface of neurons and oligodendrocytes do not exhibit localized binding in culture, and are useful primarily to identify these major cell types, particularly in mixed cultures, and to trace neuronal processes.

Other antigens are concentrated in synaptic regions *in situ*. Most of these sera bind cultured neurons in a more specific pattern (Fig. 1D). A selected sample of the binding patterns of these antibodies to frozen cerebellar sections is shown in Fig. 2, using a peroxidase reaction product to identify the location of the antigens. At this level of resolution, antibodies specific for antigens localized to terminals in the molecular layer bind numerous small punctate areas. Reaction product depositions in the granule cell layer either fill the large terminals in that layer or are deposited in thin lines surrounding them. Antibody 303 in Fig. 2A binds an antigen that fills the large terminals in the granule layer and small terminals in the molecular layer. The antigen defined by antibody 311 in Fig. 2B appears to only fill the large terminals in the granule layer,

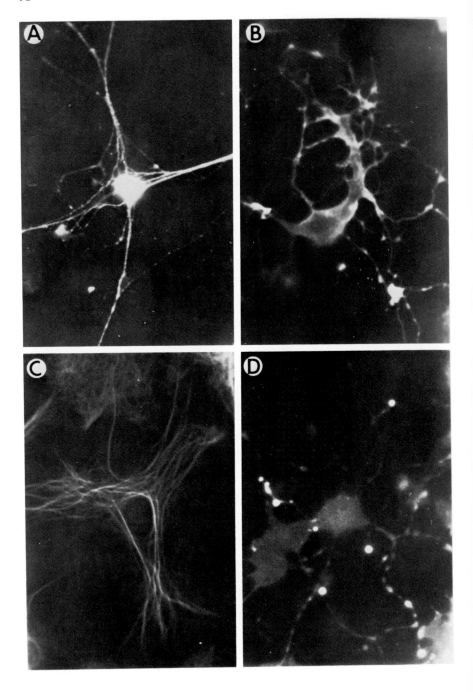

Table I. General Properties of Antigens[a]

(a) Antigen location	(b) Number of clones	(c) Representative clone number	(d) % Synaptosomes with antigen	(e) Maximum Ab binding	(f) Ratio of junction to brain binding
Neuronal surface	many	3	76	10	2.8
Oligodendrocyte surface	2	9	27	16	0.9
Astrocyte + fibroblast intermediate filaments	many	17	—	3	1.9
Mitochondria	5	201	—	—	—
Synaptic vesicle	7	48	19	5	2.1
Vesicle + postsynaptic density	1	205	—	—	—
Terminal surface	4	204	—	—	—
Not known	5	211	—	—	—

[a] Different hybridoma cultures were assigned numbers and grouped according to the location of their antigens. Column (a) lists the locations of different antigens as determined by EM immunohisto-chemistry and indirect immunofluorescense on dissociated cells in culture. The various cell types were identified by counterstaining with purified tetanus toxin for neurons, anti-GFAP for astrocytes, anti-galactocerebroside for oligodendrocytes, anti-Thy 1 for fibroblasts, and anti-RAN 1 for Schwann cells (Raff et al., 1979). Surface and internal antigens were distinguished by staining living and methanol fixed cultures. Synaptic vesicle antibodies bind to permeabilized neurons and stain neurite varicosities and terminals. Other procedures described later in this paper demonstrate that these antibodies bind synaptic vesicles. The "unknown" clones are all specific for synaptic regions at the level of resolution of the light microscope. Column (b) lists the number of clones in each class (very large in some cases). Column (c) lists representative clone numbers. In column (d) we have determined the distribution of each antigen in a synaptosome preparation described by Booth and Clark (1978). Synaptosomes were prepared and adsorbed to polylysine-coated microscope slides. Unfractionated tetanus toxin contains many breakdown products which nonspecifically stick to all types of mem-branes. Using this impure tetanus toxin and rhodamine-conjugated antibodies which recognize toxin, we could estimate the number of membranous entities in a given microscope field viewed with a 63× objective. Individual slides were incubated with tetanus toxin, fixed in methanol at −20°C, incubated simultaneously with each monoclonal antibody and human anti-tetanus toxin serum and finally with fluorescein conjugated anti-mouse Ig serum and rhodamine-coupled anti-human Ig serum. A field was photographed through rhodamine optics and then fluorescein optics. Fluorescent spots were counted and the percentage of synaptosomes with antigen was recorded as [100 × number of fluorescein spots/number of rhodamine spots]. In column (e) a limiting quantity of synaptic mem-branes, prepared according to Jones and Matus (1974), was used in a radioimmune assay to determine the relative amount of each antigen. In column (f) the amount of each antigen in synaptic junctional membranes (Wang and Mahler, 1976) is compared with the amount of antigen in synaptic membranes (Jones and Matus, 1974). Both were estimated by similar radioimmune assays.

←

Figure 1. Indirect immunofluorescence showing the binding of monoclonal antibodies to primary dissociated cells in culture. A newborn dorsal root ganglia culture is shown in (A). Antibody 22 binds a proteoglycan on the surface of the neurons in this culture. Newborn cerebral cortex cultures are shown in (B) and (C). In (B) antibody 9 binds the surface of oligodendrocytes. In (C) and (D) the cells were permeabilized before antibody incubation; (C) shows that antibody 17 binds to intermediate filaments in astrocytes; (D) shows the localization of antibody 30 binding to varicosities of a pheochromocytoma (PC12) cell line.

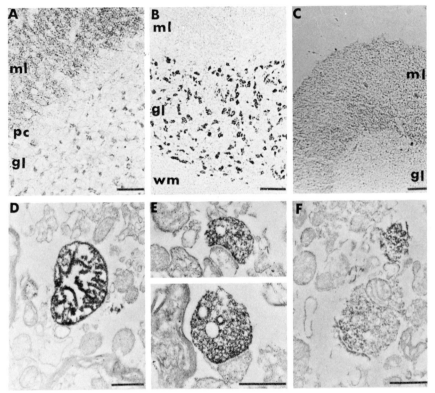

Figure 2. Examples of antibody binding to cerebellar sections and synaptosome pellets. (A, B, C) Light microscopy of 8–10-μm frozen sections of rat cerebellum incubated with different monoclonal antibodies and peroxidase-conjugated anti-mouse IgG antibodies (bar = 100 μm). Diaminobenzidine was added as a substrate for peroxidase. Reaction product appears dark. (A) The distribution of antibody 303 which binds an antigen in terminals of both the molecular and granule cell layers. (B) The antigen recognized by antibody 311 is restricted to the large terminals in the granule cell layer. (C) The binding pattern of antibody 305 which binds an antigen associated with small terminals in the molecular layer. (D, E, and F) EM photomicrographs that show the binding of antibody 302 to mitochondria (D), antibody 303 to vesicles (E), and antibody 205 to vesicles and postsynaptic densities (F) (bars = 0.5 μm). These localizations are not absolutely definitive in all cases.

while the antigen bound by antibody 305 in Fig. 2C is restricted to punctate regions in the molecular layer.

To identify the organelles bound by these antisera, we have examined binding to crude synaptosome pellets fixed after incubation with the antibodies. Antibody 302 in Fig. 2D appears to bind mitochondria; antibody 303 in Fig. 2E seems to bind synaptic vesicles; antibody 205 in

Fig. 2F binds both vesicles and postsynaptic densities. Other antibodies bind sections of plasmalemma. Antigens defined by some antibodies have not been localized with this procedure, even though the immunoperoxidase procedures do localize the antigens in frozen sections. Since these have shown very restricted binding in frozen sections (e.g., antibody 311, which is restricted to the granule cell layer in Fig. 2B), they probably bind terminals not included in this synaptosome preparation. The poor EM morphology of tissues prepared in this manner prevents definitive conclusions on localization in many cases, but does indicate which antibodies will be useful for more detailed investigation. The results do show that mitochondria and vesicles are highly concentrated in nerve terminals. The mitochondrial antigens have been detected throughout the cerebellum at lower density in fixed sections.

2.1. Characterization of Synaptosomes

One use of antibodies is to assess the purity of brain organelle preparations. The antibodies were screened against a mixed population of synaptosomes from rat brain prepared by a rapid procedure designed to preserve metabolic activities (Booth and Clark, 1978). In Table I, column d, it can be seen that neuronal surface markers bind approximately 75% of the membranous entities in such preparations, suggesting 75% are derived from neuronal material. Twenty-seven percent of the synaptosomes appear to be actually derived from myelin or oligodendrocytes, since they stain with serum 9, an oligodendrocyte marker. Only 19% of the synaptosomes contained high concentrations of a vesicle antigen. Accepting the premise, to be documented later in this paper, that this antigen is present on all or nearly all synaptic vesicles, this result argues that only 19% of these synaptosomes are actually derived from nerve terminals. A few neuronal surface markers bound very small fractions of the synaptosomes (not shown). Since they were brightly stained, this must reflect the restriction of the defined antigens to subpopulations of neurons or membranes in the synaptosome mixture. In summary, the results in Table I, column d, argue that this particular synaptosome preparation is less pure than previously believed and illustrate some of the principles by which antisera can be used to characterize biochemical preparations. Obviously, such antisera can be used to further purify organelle preparations, and one example will be presented later in this paper.

The total amount of a particular antibody that can be bound by a limiting amount of a synaptic membrane preparation differs widely (column e) and provides one means of estimating the relative amounts of the different antigens. When binding to synaptic junctions is com-

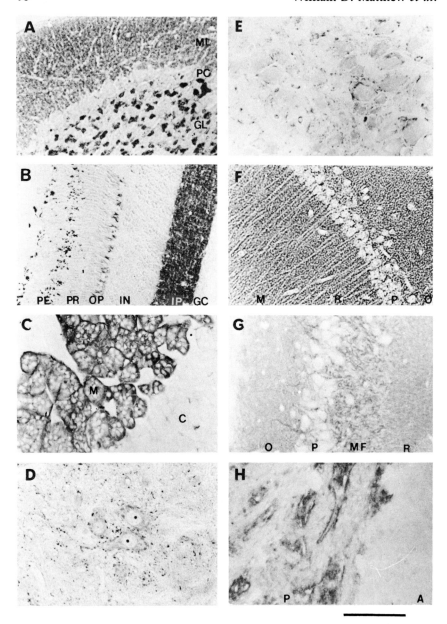

Figure 3. Immunocytochemical localization of serum 30 immunoreactivity in the nervous system. Light microscopy of representative 8–10-μm formaldehyde-fixed, frozen sections incubated with serum 30 and rat PAP complex or peroxidase conjugate are shown in this figure (bar = 100 μm). The methods have been described by Sternberger, 1979; Vaughn *et al.*, 1980. The peroxidase reaction product appears dark. Unless indicated, sections are not counterstained. (A) Rat cerebellar cortex, showing granule cell layer (GL) at bottom,

pared with binding to total brain membranes, most of the antigens are enriched in the junction preparation (column f), providing preliminary evidence that they may be preferentially localized to synapses.

3. ANTIBODIES THAT SHOW LOCALIZED BINDING IN THE BRAIN

For the rest of this paper, we will concentrate on one antibody that binds a vesicle-specific protein as an example of how monoclonal sera are characterized and applied to studies on the nervous system.

3.1. Localization of Serum 30 Immunoreactivity to Nerve Terminals

In sections of the cerebellum (Fig. 3A), using peroxidase reaction product to detect antigenic activity, serum 30 binds the large glomeruli

---

Purkinje cell layer (PC) in center, and molecular layer (ML) at top. The peroxidase reaction product is abundant in synaptic regions, staining the small synapses in the molecular layer with small punctate depositions and the large synaptic glomeruli in the granule cell layer with large reaction product depositions. The white matter (not shown) contained no reaction product. (B) Frog retina, showing the pigment epithelium (PE) at the left, the photoreceptors (PR), outer nuclear layer (not abbreviated), outer plexiform layer (OP), inner nuclear layer (IN), inner plexiform layer (IP), and ganglion cells (GC). Peroxidase product is seen in the two synaptic layers—the outer and inner plexiform layers. The dark product in the pigment epithelium is endogenous melanin and is seen in control sections. Although not apparent in black and white photographs, the two deposits are easily distinguishable, since the melanin is black and the peroxidase product is brown. (C) Rat adrenal gland, showing the medulla (M) and cortex (C). Peroxidase reaction product is seen in the medulla but not the cortex. (D) Rat thoracic spinal cord, showing the large motoneurons in the ventral gray matter. This section was lightly counterstained with toluidine blue to reveal the motoneuron somas. Reaction product in the axosomatic synapses on the motoneurons is particularly dramatic. (E) Frog paravertebral sympathetic ganglion (T9 or T10), showing the large principal sympathetic neuron cell somas. Peroxidase reaction product is localized to punctate areas between the cell somas, as is expected in this ganglion where the majority of synapses are formed on dendrites. The light brown coloring of the cell somas was also seen in controls. (F) Rat hippocampus, CA1 area, showing the stratum moleculare (M) at the left, the stratum radiatum (R), stratum pyramidale (P), and stratum oriens (O). Many different types of synapses are found between cells in these areas, and punctate depositions of peroxidase reaction product are also seen throughout the section. (G) Rat hippocampus, CA3 area, showing the stratum oriens (O) at the left, stratum pyramidale (P), mossy fiber terminals (MF), and stratum radiatum (R). Small depositions of reaction product, corresponding to the synaptic terminals, are found throughout this section. Somewhat larger 3- to 6-μm terminals, formed by mossy fibers, and correspondingly larger depositions of reaction product, are found in the mossy fiber area (MF). (H) Rabbit pituitary, showing portions of the posterior (P) and anterior (A) lobes. Peroxidase reaction product is evident in the posterior lobe in regions surrounding the capillaries.

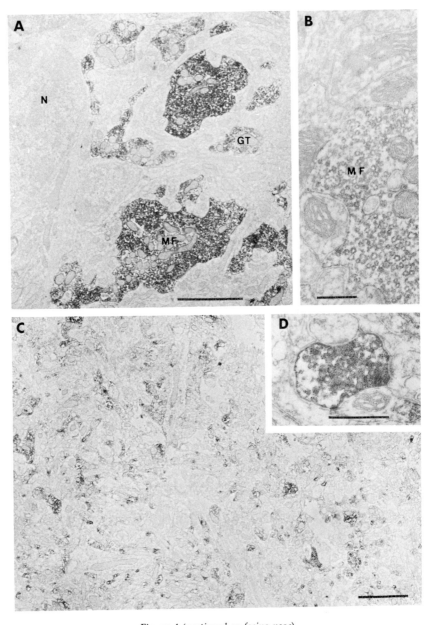

Figure 4 (*continued on facing page*).

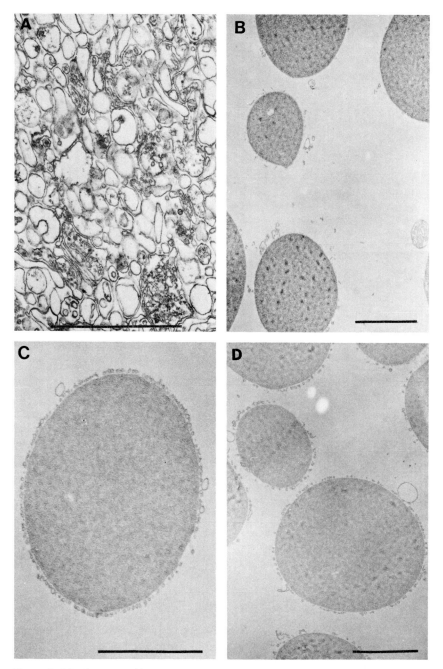

Figure 5. Membrane profiles immunoprecipitated on protein-A–acrylamide beads. An electron micrograph of a sectioned crude brain homogenate is shown in (A); an electron micrograph of a sectioned acrylamide bead with attached membrane profiles immunoprecipitated with normal mouse serum is shown in (B). In (C) and (D) are profiles precipitated with serum 30 (all bars = 1 μm). General procedures are described by Ito and Palade (1978).

chondria, vesicles, and debris. This mixture was incubated with normal mouse serum or serum 30 and precipitated after mixing with polyacrylamide beads coupled to protein A. Only an occasional piece of membrane was found on the surface of the polyacrylamide beads when control serum was used (Fig. 5B). Even cleaner profiles of beads were seen when a monoclonal antiserum against intermediate filaments was used as a control (not shown). In contrast, large numbers of profiles with the same size as synaptic vesicles are precipitated on the surface of the acrylamide beads after incubation with serum 30 (Fig. 5C,D). Mitochondrial profiles are absent. We have tabulated the structures seen in sections of serum 30 precipitates and starting nerve terminal lysates in Table II. The amount of nonvesicular material is reduced 30-fold by this single step. The presence of the vesicle antigen is inverted vesicles of surface membrane limits the efficiency of this procedure, but homogenization in the absence of Ca^{2+}, homogenization after rapid freezing, and separation in molecular seive columns should reduce or eliminate this contamination (cf. Carlson *et al.*, 1978).

To demonstrate that the vesicles isolated by this procedure still contained their internal contents, we incubated PC12 cells with [^{3}H]NE prior to homogenization and immunoprecipitation. The data in Table III estimate the efficiency with which [^{3}H]NE is retained in the vesicles during the incubation with antiserum and other manipulations by measuring the efficiency of [^{3}H] retention on millipore filters, which previous investigators (cf. Patterson *et al.*, 1975) have shown retain vesicular, but not cytoplasmic, NE. Ninety-five percent of the [^{3}H]NE remaining in vesicles could be precipitated by the antiserum, so immunoprecipitation of vesicles and their internal contents appears to be very efficient. Ef-

Table II. Selective Immunoprecipitation of Synaptic Vesicles with Serum 30[a]

	Vesicles	Other profiles	Total profiles	Ratio of vesicles to other profiles
Crude homogenate	136	1165	1301	0.12
Profiles precipitated with serum 30	1357	376	1733	3.61

[a] The profiles seen in electron micrographs of lysed crude brain homogenate (cf. Fig. 4A) and a membrane fraction purified by immunoprecipitation (cf. Fig. 4C, D) are tabulated. Only profiles that could be unambiguously identified as synaptic vesicles were counted in that category. These results are the average of two separate experiments that did not differ significantly from each other.

Table III. Efficiency of Immunoprecipitation of [³H]-
Norepinephrine[a]

	Total CPM	CPM on filter	CPM on beads
Cell homogenate, time 0	5200	2100	—
Cell homogenate, time 4 hr	5200	940	—
Cell homogenate, time 4 hr with serum 30	5200	980	930

[a] 10^6 PC12 cells were incubated with 1 μCi [³H]NE for 80 min at 37°C (Patterson et al., 1975). Cells were homogenized in 1 ml of growth medium with a glass–teflon homogenizer. Then large debris was removed by centrifugation at 10,000 g for 5 min. Aliquots were used to estimate the vesicular [³H]NE content by millipore filtration (Patterson et al., 1975). Preparations were incubated at room temperature and samples removed and adsorbed to millipore filters to determine the rate at which transmitter leaks out of these vesicles. Values are cited for 4 hr, the time required to complete the immunoprecipitation on beads. Aliquots were used for immunoprecipitations: 300-μl aliquots were mixed with 40 μg of each antibody, incubated for 100 min at 2°C, and adsorbed to immobilize protein A.

ficiency could undoubtedly be improved by shortening the incubation times and adjusting reagent concentrations.

3.3. Widespread Distribution of the Antigenic Determinant(s) in Neurosecretory Tissues

Antigenic competition assays provide a method for quantitating the amounts of particular antigens more rigorously than is possible with immunohistochemical procedures, although they lack the resolution of the latter methods. We used such an assay to measure the concentration of vesicle antigen in different parts of the nervous system, in nonneural secretory organs, in nonsecretory tissues, and in cell lines derived from tumors that developed in these different organs. The results in Table IV show that the serum 30 determinant(s) is found in every part of the central or peripheral nervous system tested, including cerebral and cerebellar cortices, midbrain, posterior pituitary, adrenal medulla, and superior cervical ganglion. In contrast, the concentration in two nonsecretory tissues—noninnervated muscle and adrenal cortex—was below the detection limits of the assay. Significantly higher levels of antigen were seen in nonneural secretory tissues, such as the liver, pancreas, and salivary gland, but the levels were low enough that it seems possible they reflect the known presence of nerve terminals in these organs, not concentrations of antigen in the endogenous secretory cells. The antigenic determinants are found, however, both in the anterior pituitary and two cell lines—AtT20 and GH3—derived from that tissue at low but significant concentrations, so the antigen(s) must exist in this non-neural secretory tissue.

To summarize, at the level of resolution provided by the light microscope, the antigen(s) appears to be present in every visible synaptic layer of those portions of the nervous system that have been examined (Figs. 2 and 3), including cerebellum, retina, spinal cord, hippocampus, sympathetic ganglion, and pituitary. The antigen is present in putative glutaminergic and GABAnergic terminals (cerebellar parallel fibers and Golgi type II endings), catecholaminergic tissue (adrenal, PC12), sero-

Table IV. Quantitative Measurement of Antigen[a]

Material homogenized	% RSA
Tissues	
Extrajunctional diaphragm muscle (rabbit)	<0.3
Adrenal cortex (bovine)	<0.4
Pancreas (rabbit)	0.9
Liver (rabbit)	0.9
Salivary gland (rabbit)	5.4
Anterior pituitary (bovine)	11
Superior cervical ganglion (rabbit)	27
Adrenal medulla (bovine)	76
Posterior pituitary (bovine)	86
Cerebral cortex (rabbit)	75
Cerebellum (rabbit)	60
Superior colliculus (rabbit)	50
Whole brain (rat)	100
Cell types	% RSA
Blood cells (rabbit)	<.2
HIT (hamster pancreatic islet)	<.05
AtT20 (mouse anterior pituitary)	5.0
GH3 (rat anterior pituitary)	12
PC12 (rat adrenal phaeochromocytoma)	26
PC12 grown in NGF	38

[a] Aliquots of 76 ng/ml of ascites fluid 48 in 5% newborn calf serum in PBS (a dilution chosen to be limiting in the assay) were incubated with different concentrations of homogenized tissues for 12 hr at 4°C. The membranes were pelleted at 200,000g for 40 min in an airfuge. The residual antibody in the supernatant was measured in the solid-phase radioimmune assay (Klinman, 1972). The amount of tissue protein needed to adsorb 50% of the binding was recorded from inhibiton curves. The inverse values were normalized to rat brain defined as 100% relative specific activity (RSA). (A % relative specific activity equals $\left[\dfrac{\text{(antigen units/mg tissue)}}{\text{(antigen units/mg adult rat brain)}} \right] \times 100$).

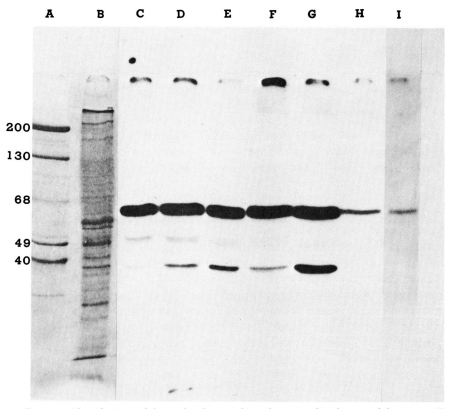

Figure 6. Identification of the molecular weight and species distribution of the serum 30 antigen(s). A portion of a whole brain was dissolved in SDS–mercaptoethanol and processed as described by Burridge (1978). Gel lanes containing protein standards and rat brain, both stained with Coomassie blue, are shown at the left (lanes A and B). The molecular manner of the protein standards in kilodaltons are indicated. The different species used as sources for the brain homogenates were rat (C), mouse (D), rabbit (E), cow (F), chicken (G), frog (H), and shark (I).

tonergic tissue (pineal), and cholinergic cells or endings (PC12, presynaptic terminals in sympathetic ganglion). It is also found in a variety of peptidergic cells or terminals [the LHRH terminals in the frog sympathetic ganglion (L. Y. Jan and N. Jan, personal communication), growth-hormone-secreting GH3 cells, ACTH- and endorphin-releasing AtT20 cells, and posterior and anterior pituitary (Table IV)]. We are left with the conclusion that this protein is very widely distributed in synaptic vesicles and may be present in every type of neuronal terminal.

3.4. Molecular-Weight and Evolutionary Distribution of the Antigen(s)

To determine the specificity of the antiserum, we denatured a brain homogenate in boiling SDS and separated the denatured proteins by molecular weight on an acrylamide gel (Laemmli, 1970). After separation, antibody molecules were diffused into the gel and the molecular weight of the antigen(s) was determined (Burridge, 1978). In Fig. 6, one can see that serum 30 binds a 65,000-dalton protein found in shark, chicken, frog, and every mammal tested. Clearly the antigen has persisted through several hundred million years of evolutionary divergence. The autoradiograph of the gel in Fig. 6 was intentionally overexposed to emphasize the comparatively small amount of antibody binding to two bands at 40,000 and 50,000 daltons that is invisible in shorter exposures that reveal the 65,000-dalton protein. We suspect that these two minor bands are proteolytic fragments of the 65,000-dalton protein. If so, the protease-sensitive sites must have been preserved in the different species, since the same-sized fragments are always observed. This suggests that the major features of the protein are highly conserved. When the amounts of antigen in the brains of the different species were measured, using the same immune competition assay described in Table IV, comparable levels were seen in every vertebrate listed in Fig. 6 (70–200% of the amount in homogenized rat brain, data not shown).

4. SUMMARY AND DISCUSSION

We have isolated a series of monoclonal antibodies that distinguish the major cell types of the nervous system and recognize molecules concentrated at synapses. Characterization of other antisera is continuing in the laboratory. In evaluating our past experience, we have found that solid-phase radioimmune assays in microtiter plates have not provided reliable information on the localization of particularly antigens in the brain and speculate that this may reflect differences in the efficiency with which different antigens adhere to polyvinylchloride plastic. Immune competition assays are reliable, but much more tedious. In general, immunohistochemical procedures have provided the most reliable information and are now being done routinely in initial screens.

The antibodies described in this paper have been used to characterize the purity of a brain synaptosome preparation. Similar antisera should prove invaluable in the future in assaying the efficacy of purification schemes for different cell types or organelles. One antiserum, which binds the outside of synaptic vesicles, has been used to purify these organelles efficiently with their transmitter contents. This antiserum should be useful for identifying unknown transmitter substances or for verifying that putative transmitters are indeed contained within synaptic vesicles. The antiserum also shows that many different types of neurosecretory vesicles share at least one common vesicle-specific protein, a relationship whose basis is probably in a common function, preservation of which has blocked significant evolutionary divergence in the millions of years of vertebrate speciation. The protein is integrally, not peripherally associated with vesicle membranes. It does not correspond to protein I or the various cytoskeletal proteins hypothesized to be associated with synaptic vesicles (cf. Bloom *et al.*, 1979; Meyer and Burger, 1979), but it could be one of the protein bands detected on acrylamide gels in synaptic vesicle fractions (cf. Wagner and Kelly, 1979). Its function is not currently known and will be a challenging biochemical detection problem.

A family of antibodies is directed against neuronal surface molecules, many of which appear to be proteoglycans containing very large carbohydrate residues. One of these antigens has been shown to have a distinctly different distribution *in culture* and *in situ,* suggesting that substrate interactions are important for governing the secretion or storage of these molecules. Similar interactions have already been shown to be important for promoting and guiding neuronal growth (cf. Rutishauser and Edelman, 1980) and synapse formation (cf. Sanes *et al.*, 1978). We are currently using the localization of these synapse-associated molecules in assays to detect and purify the endogenous factors required for synaptogenesis by motoneurons and other cells in the nervous system.

ACKNOWLEDGMENTS

We thank our colleagues at UCSF, especially Drs. Regis Kelly and Allan Basbaum, for discussions and help with methodological problems. We also thank Liz Neville and Veronica Oliva for their patience in typing the manuscript. Research was supported by grants to LFR from the National Science Foundation, Muscular Dystrophy Association, McKnight Foundation, March of Dimes Birth Defects Foundation, and Wills Foundation. LFR is a Sloan Foundation Fellow.

5. REFERENCES

Bloom, F. E., Ueda, T., Battenberg, E., and Greengard, P., 1979, Immunocytochemical localization in synapses of protein I, an endogenous substrate for protein kinases in mammalian brain, *Proc. Natl. Acad. Sci. U.S.A.* **76**:5982.

Booth, R. F. G., and Clark, J. B., 1978, A rapid method for the preparation of relatively pure metabolically competent synaptosomes from rat brain, *Biochem. J.* **176**:365.

Burridge, K., 1978, Direct identification of specific glycoproteins and antigens in SDS gels, *Methods Enzymol.* **50**:54.

Carlin, R. K., Grab, D. J., Cohen, R. S., and Siekevitz, P., 1980, Isolation and characterization of postsynaptic densities from various brain regions: Enrichment of different types of postsynaptic densities, *J. Cell Biol.* **86**:831.

Carlson, S. S., Wagner, J. A., and Kelly, R. B., 1978, Purification of synaptic vesicles from Elasmobranch Electric Organ and the use of biophysical criteria to demonstrate purity, *Biochemistry* **17**:1188.

Heuser, J. E., 1978, Synaptic vesicle exocytosis and recycling during transmitter discharge from the neuromuscular junction, in: *Transport of Macromolecules in Cellular Systems* (S. C. Silverstein, ed.), pp. 445–464, Dahlem Konferenzen, Berlin.

Hildebrand, J., Barker, D., Herbert, E., and Kravitz, E., 1971, Screening for neurotransmitters—A rapid radiochemical procedure, *J. Neurobiol.* **2**:231.

Hokfelt, T., Johansson, O., Ljungdahl, A., Lundberg, J. M., and Schultzberg, M., 1980, Peptidergic neurons, *Nature (London)* **284**:515.

Ito, A., and Palade, G., 1978, Presence of NADPH-cytochrome P-450 veductase in rat liver golgi membranes; Evidence obtained by immunoabsorption method, *J. Cell Biol.* **79**:590.

Jones, D. H., and Matus, A. I., 1974, Isolation of synaptic plasma membranes from brain by combined flotation-sedimentation density gradient centrifugation, *Biochem. Biophys. Acta* **356**:276.

Klinman, N. R., 1972, The mechanism of antigenic stimulation of primary and secondary clonal precursor cells, *J. Exp. Med.* **136**:241.

Laemmli, U. K., 1970, Cleavage of structural proteins during the assembly of the head of bacteriophage T4. *Nature (London)* **227**:680.

Mahler, H., 1977, Proteins of the synaptic membrane, *Neurochem. Res.* **2**:119.

Matus, A., and Taff-Jones, D., 1978, Morphology and molecular composition of isolated postsynaptic junctional structures, *Proc. R. Soc. London Ser. B* **203**:135.

Meyer, D. I., and Burger, M. M., 1979, The chromaffin granule surface—The presence of actin and the nature of its interaction with the membrane, *FEBS Lett.* **101**:129.

Patterson, P. H., Reichardt, L. F., and Chun, L. L. Y., 1975, Biochemical studies on the development of primary sympathetic neurons in cell culture, *Cold Spring Harbor Symp. Quant. Biol.* **15**:389.

Raff, M., Fields, K. L., Hakamori, S., Mirsky, R., Pruss, R. M., and Winter, J., 1979, Cell type-specific markers for distinguishing and studying neurons and the major classes of glial cells in culture, *Brain Res.* **174**:283.

Rutishauser, U., and Edelman, G. M., 1980, Effects of fasciculation on the outgrowth of neurites from spinal ganglia in culture. *J. Cell Biol.* **87**:370.

Sanes, J. R., Marshall, L., and McMahan, U. J., 1978, Reinnervation of muscle fiber basal lamina after removal of myofibers, *J. Cell Biol.* **78**:176.

Stell, W., Marshak, D., Yamada, T., Brecha, N., and Karten, H., 1980, Peptides are in the eye of the beholder, *Trends Neurosci.* **3**:292.

Sternberger, L. A., 1979, Immunocytochemistry, 2nd ed., Wiley, New York.

Vaughn, J. E., Barber, R. P., Ribuk, C. E., and Houser, C. R., 1980, Methods for the immunocytochemical localization of protein and peptides involved in neurotransmission, in: *Current Trends in Morphological Technique* vol. 3 (J. J. Johnson, ed.) CRC Press, Boca Raton, Fla.

Wagner, J. A., and Kelly, R. B., 1979, Topological organization of proteins in an intracellular secretory organelle: The synaptic vesicle, *Proc. Natl. Acad. Sci. U.S.A.* **76**:4126.

Wang, Y.-J., and Mahler, H. R., 1976, Topography of the synaptosomal membrane, *J. Cell Biol.* **71**:639.

Wood, J. G., McLaughlin, B. J., and Vaughn, J. E., 1976, Immunocytochemical localization of GAD in EM preparations of rodent CNS, in: *GABA in Nervous System Function*, Roberts, Chase, and Tower, eds., pp. 133–148, Raven Press, N.Y.

Wood, J. G., Wallace, R. W., Whittaker, J. N., and Cheung, W. Y., 1980, Immunocytochemical localization of calmoldulin and a heat-labile calmodulin binding protein (CaM-BP$_{80}$) in basal ganglia of mouse brain, *J. Cell Biol.* **84**:66.

4

Analysis of Functional Cell Sets in the Immune System

LINDA L. Y. CHUN and HARVEY CANTOR

In the immune system it has been possible to distinguish subpopulations of cells on the basis of the surface antigens they express. The genetic program of each set of cells combines information which codes for a unique pattern of cell surface glycoproteins that is invariably associated with a particular immunologic function. More recently, it has been possible to identify the functional role of one of these surface glycoproteins. The purpose of this article is to review the experimental approaches which have contributed to the definition of functional cell sets in the immune system in the hope that similar strategies may be useful in the dissection of functionally relevant cell sets in the nervous system.

The cellular elements important for immune function are macrophages and lymphocytes. Macrophages, which are found in all tissues of the body, accumulate foreign substances and present them to lymphocytes. Lymphocytes, which circulate throughout the body, are directly responsible for specific immune responses. There are two major classes of lymphocytes: (1) the T lymphocytes or T cells, which develop in the thymus, and (2) the B lymphocytes or B cells, which develop in the bone marrow. The type of immune response and its intensity generated by antigen stimulation are regulated by interactions among these cells.

LINDA L. Y. CHUN and HARVEY CANTOR   Department of Pathology, Harvard Medical School, and Sidney Farber Cancer Institute, Boston, Mass.

In this article we will focus on T lymphocytes. Despite their uniform morphology, T cells do not form a homogeneous population; in fact, they mediate a wide variety of immunologic functions. In one type of function, called helper function, T cells assist B cells to produce antibody (Claman *et al.*, 1966; Miller and Mitchell, 1968). A second type of function, called suppressor function, was discovered in studies of immunologic tolerance. These studies showed that T cells from an animal that did not produce antibodies in response to a given antigen, when transferred to a normal animal, made it unable to produce antibodies (Gershon, 1974). In a third type of function, called cytotoxic or killer function, T cells destroy foreign grafts or cells which are made antigenically foreign by virus infection or malignant transformation (Cantor and Asofsky, 1972). To understand immune regulation it is important to determine how this heterogeneity of T-cell function is generated. Either these functions are mediated by a single set of pluripotential T cells whose choice of function is governed by the mode or type of antigen stimulation, or alternatively, they are mediated by different subsets of T cells genetically programmed during differentiation to express only one of these functions.

1. T-CELL SETS

This would be resolved if T cells from unimmunized animals could be subdivided into different sets which when stimulated by antigen would make only one of the possible T-cell responses. It was necessary to find a technique which would permit identification as well as separation of relevant T-cell subclasses. The development by Boyse and his colleagues (1968, 1971) of alloantisera which defined a panel of cell surface differentiation antigens, the Lyt antigens, on mouse thymocytes and some peripheral lymphocytes provided the basis. Since these components were not detected on cells of other tissues (brain, kidney, liver, epidermal cells, B lymphocytes, or bone marrow), they seemed to represent components specified by genes expressed exclusively during T-cell differentiation. The Lyt antigens discussed here include Lyt-1, Lyt-2, and Lyt-3. Each of the Lyt loci is expressed as one of two alleles which permitted the generation of specific alloantisera. The Lyt-1 glycoprotein is coded for by a gene on chromosome 19, and the Lyt-2 and Lyt-3 components are both coded for by genes on chromosome 6 (Itakura *et al.*, 1972). With the use of antisera or monoclonal antibodies against the Lyt antigens, these glycoproteins, immunoprecipitated from thymocytes, have been biochemically analyzed. Anti-Lyt-1 antisera precipitates two polypeptides with extreme charge heterogeneity and apparent molecular weights of 67,000 and 87,000 (Durda *et al.*, 1978; Ledbetter and Herzenberg, 1979). The Lyt-2 and Lyt-3 determinants are on different, but very basic, polypeptide subunits, which are associated covalently in molecular complexes by disulfide bonds. Anti-Lyt-2 antibodies precipitate two subunits with apparent molecular weights of 34,000 and 38,000, whereas anti-Lyt-3 antibodies precipitate only one polypeptide, with apparent molecular weight of 30,000 (Reilly *et al.*, 1980; Ledbetter *et al.*, 1981).

The experimental approach used was to eliminate different sets of T cells with the use of alloantisera against each of the Lyt antigens and then test the remainder for various T-cell functions. For example, lymphocytes which express the Lyt-1 surface antigen are lysed when exposed to antisera against Lyt-1 in the presence of complement (Cantor and Boyse, 1975*a*). The lysis is monitored with trypan blue, which stains lysed but not live cells, or by the release of a radioactive label from the lysed cells. Alternatively, cells which express surface Lyt-1 can be positively selected on columns or plates coated with anti-Lyt-1 antisera. The crucial aspect to this approach is the ability to generate *specific* alloantisera against the Lyt components (Shen *et al.*, 1975). More recently, this problem has been circumvented through the use of monoclonal antibodies. These subsets are then tested for ability to mediate cytolysis, help B cells secrete antibody, or induce lymphocyte proliferation.

These studies have indicated that the peripheral T-cell pool contains at least three separate T-cell sets (Table I): the Lyt-123 set, the Lyt-1 set, and the Lyt-23 set. They compose, respectively, 50%, 30%, and approximately 5–10% of the peripheral T-cell pool. Thus, according to the

Table I. Properties of T Lymphocyte Sets

Cell surface phenotype[a]	Function
Lyt-1 cell set (Thy-1$^+$, Lyt-1$^+$, Lyt-2$^-$, Lyt-3$^-$)	Induce or activate effector cells (suppressor T cells, cytotoxic T cells, mast cells, basophils, monocytes, eosinophils) to fulfill their respective genetic programs
Lyt-23 cell set (Thy-1$^+$, Lyt-1$^-$, Lyt-2$^+$, Lyt-3$^+$)	Suppressor T cells suppress immune responses Cytotoxic T cells kill antigenically foreign cells
Lyt-123 cell set (Thy-1$^+$, Lyt-1$^+$, Lyt-2$^+$, Lyt-3$^+$)	Precursor of T inducer cells Precursor of T effector cells Amplifier cells Feedback suppressor cells

[a] Each of these cell sets undoubtedly will be and in some cases has already been shown to be further divisible into subsets with the use of other cell surface markers.

criterion of selective expression of gene products on the cell surface, the T-cell pool is divisible into at least three groups of cells, each following a different set of genetic instructions. In addition, these individual differentiative programs include information that decides what the function of each T-cell set should be.

Cells of the Lyt-1 set are genetically programmed to help or amplify the activity of other cells after stimulation by antigen. These cells are called inducer cells since they will induce or activate other cell sets to fulfill their respective genetic programs: Lyt-1 cells induce (1) B cells to secrete antibody (Cantor and Boyse, 1975a), (2) macrophages and monocytes to participate in delayed-type hypersensitivity responses (Huber et al., 1976), and (3) precursors of killer cells to differentiate into killer–effector cells (Cantor and Boyse, 1975a). More recently, Lyt-1 cells have been found to induce a set of resting, nonimmune T cells to generate potent feedback-suppresive activity (Eardley et al., 1978; Cantor et al., 1978). Analysis of isolated Lyt-1 inducer cells from nonimmune donors indicates that these cells are already programmed for helper/inducer function before overt immunization with antigen; this function is independent of the ability of Lyt-1 inducer cells to interact with antigen (Jandinski et al., 1976; Cantor et al., 1976).

In contrast, cells of the Lyt-23 set are specially equipped both to develop alloreactive cytotoxic activity as well as to suppress both humoral and cell-mediated immune responses following immunization (Cantor and Boyse, 1975a,b; Jandinski et al., 1976). Whether cytotoxicity and antigen-induced suppression are two manifestations of one genetic program or whether they represent the phenotype of two separate genetic programs is not yet clearly established. However, at least some cells in the Lyt-23 suppressor set express a surface antigen coded for in the I-J subregion of the major histocompatibility complex (Murphy, 1978). This gene product has not been found on cytotoxic cells or their precursors. This suggests that although similar in many characteristics, mature killer and suppressor cells are separable.

Cells of the Lyt-123 phenotype have been the least well defined of the various T-cell sets. The most likely possibility is that at least some of these cells represent a store of intermediary cells that regulate the supply and function of more mature Lyt-1 and Lyt-23 cells. This is based in part on experiments which show that (1) after stimulation with chemically altered syngeneic cells, some Lyt-123 cells give rise to Lyt-23 progeny (Finberg et al., 1978), and (2) purified populations of Lyt-123 cells can give rise to Lyt-1 cells after mitogenic activation by concanavalin A.

More recently, it has been demonstrated that resting Lyt-123 cells can be induced by antigen-stimulated Lyt-1 cells to develop profound feedback-suppressive activity. The term *feedback* is used since the degree of suppressive activity exerted by a fixed number of nonimmune Lyt-123 cells increases in direct proportion to the number of antigen-activated Lyt-1 cells in the system (Eardley *et al.*, 1978), and one target of the suppression is the inducer Lyt-1 cell itself. These results indicate that, as with the formation of antibody, the generation of immunologic suppression after stimulation by antigen also requires induction by Lyt-1 cells. There are most assuredly as yet unidentified sets of T cells which exhibit different cell surface glycoproteins and mediate other T-cell functions. These will no doubt be identified as new genetically defined surface antigens are discovered and/or with the use of T-cell clone technology (see below).

2. FUNCTIONAL ROLES FOR Lyt ANTIGENS

In the preceding section we saw that T cells with different functions can be distinguished on the basis of their expression of Lyt antigens. Do these antigens play a direct role in T-cell function? Thus far, the best evidence that Lyt antigens contribute directly to T-cell function comes from studies of cytotoxic T lymphocytes. These cells express Lyt-23 on their surface and kill antigenically foreign cells by inducing their lysis. To examine the role of Lyt-2 in this process, the ability of cytotoxic T cells to kill target cells was assessed in the presence of antibodies to Lyt-2 in the absence of complement. The effect of both alloantisera (Nakayama *et al.*, 1979; Shinohara and Sachs, 1979) and monoclonal antibodies (Hollander, *et al.*, 1980; Sarmiento *et al.*, 1980) to Lyt-2 was to specifically block the ability of cytotoxic T cells to kill target cells. No blocking was observed with antisera against other cell surface alloantigens such as TL, Thy-1, H-2, or immunoglobulin determinants. These studies establish a role for Lyt-2 in cytotoxic T-cell function but do not define its mechanism of action. Some insight to this is provided by work with a cloned cytotoxic T-cell line, L3 (Glasebrook and Fitch, 1980). L3 specifically lyses targets that express on their surface H-2D^d alloantigen. However, L3 will lyse targets which do not express H-2D^d, if stimulated by Con A, a nonspecific mitogen. Variants of this L3 line, which lack Lyt-2 and Lyt-3 on their surface, cannot kill H-2D^d target cells except in the presence of Con A (Dialynas *et al.*, 1981). These results suggest that Lyt-2 is involved in the antigen recognition rather than the cell lysis step. Thus, Lyt-2 is a cell surface differentiation antigen which not only identifies a subset of T cells but also plays a direct role in its cytotoxic function. In addition, Hollander *et al.* (1980) found that monoclonal antibodies against Lyt-2 in the absence of complement will also inhibit alloantigen-induced T-cell proliferation and generation of killer cells. As with the variant experiments, in contrast to alloantigen-induced stimulation, Con-A-induced T-cell proliferation was not inhibited by anti-Lyt-2. This again suggests that for T-cell proliferation, as with cytolytic T-cell function, Lyt-2 is important at the level of antigen recognition.

Finally, recent experiments by Hollander et al. (1981) suggest a possible role for Lyt-1. In the absence of complement, monoclonal antibody against Lyt-1 stimulates cell proliferation and generation of cytotoxic T cells in mixed lymphocyte cultures by causing an increase in the production of T-cell growth factors (TCGF). The cellular circuit which mediates this response is not yet clear. Anti-Lyt-1 could stimulate a set of Lyt-1 inducer cells which produce TCGF, or alternatively, it could inhibit a set of Lyt-1 suppressor cells, which inhibits TCGF production.

Thus, this cellular approach to the study of immune regulation has produced the current view that the immune system is composed of sets of functionally different cells: inducer, regulatory, and effector cells. Each cell set expresses as part of its genetic program a characteristic set of surface glycoproteins or differentiation antigens, which also determines the function of the set and at least in the case of Lyt-2 is also involved directly in the execution of that function. When the system is stimulated by antigen, the intensity of the immune response depends on the relative degree of activation of these various sets. If the net effect is excitatory, immunity results and, for example, T cells induce B cells to produce antibody against antigen. On the other hand, when the net effect is inhibitory, suppression results, and T suppressor cells inactivate T cells that induce B cells to secrete antibody. Thus, the ability to prevent immune responses against an animal's own tissues depends not on the elimination at birth of cell sets which recognize these tissues but on active suppression of these sets throughout the life of the animal.

3. T-CELL CLONES

Thus far, analysis of the cell sets which form the immune system has shown that Lyt antigens are extremely useful for the definition of functional cell sets and also play a direct role in antigen-specific function. T-cell sets genetically defined by these differentiation antigens can induce or suppress antibody formation. It is important to understand the molecular basis of these specific interactions. Examination of specific T-cell sets indicates that soluble factors can mimic the functions of intact T suppressor or T inducer cells (Takemori and Tada, 1975; Mozes and

Haimovich, 1979). However, it has been difficult to examine the structural basis of antigen-specific T-cell function. This is probably due to the fact that uncloned T-cell populations, obtained by negative selection using antibodies against surface molecules and complement, contain small numbers of contaminating cells which often complicate interpretation of biochemical and functional data. Thus, definition of the molecular basis of cellular interactions will be facilitated by large numbers of homogeneous T cells.

Recently, it has become technically feasible to generate homogeneous populations of antigen-specific inducer or suppressor T cells, which arise from clonal expansion of cells at discrete steps of differentiation. To achieve this it was important to clone cells before *in vitro* expansion, because in populations of unseparated T cells, inducer cells specifically activate suppressor cells. Since one target of activated suppressor cells is the inducer cell itself, there is a loss of antigen-specific suppressor cell activity in heterogeneous cultures. In addition, different culture conditions must be defined for each T-cell clone to support long-term clonal expansion without loss of function. All the Lyt-1^+2^- clones obtained so far mediate inducer but not suppressor activity and synthesize a characteristic pattern of polypeptides. In contrast, Lyt-2^+ clones mediate suppressor but not inducer activity and synthesize a characteristic set of proteins that differs from T inducer cells (Nabel *et al.*, 1981).

One of these T suppressor clones expresses the Lyt-2 surface marker and inhibits antibody response to sheep red blood cells (SRBC). This clone synthesizes a glycoprotein of 70,000 molecular weight which specifically binds to SRBC and can suppress the formation of antibody against SRBC (Fresno *et al.*, 1981a,b). Biochemical analysis of this molecule has provided important information on the structural basis of antigen-specific suppression. Fresno *et al.* (1982) found that papain splits the T suppressor glycoprotein into two fragments of 45,000 and 24,000 molecular weight. Examination of the biologic activity of these peptides indicated that the 45,000 fragment retains antigen-independent suppressor activity. In contrast, the 24,000 fragment binds specifically to SRBC but does not suppress the antibody response. Thus, the suppressor factor has two functional domains mediated by different parts of the molecule. This is reminiscent of papain digestion of the immunoglobulin molecule, which also produces two fragments, Fc and Fab. The Fc fragment carries the biologic activity of different immunoglobulin subclasses, whereas the Fab fragment carries the antigen binding site (Edelman, 1971; Natvig and Kunkel, 1973).

What implications do these studies have for our understanding of nervous system function? Can a particular cell surface differentiation antigen be correlated with a subset of neuronal synapses mediating a particular function? One possibility is as follows: physiologic inhibition is often mediated by channels which permit passage of ions, such as K^+ or Cl^-, whose equilibrium potentials lie below threshold (Coombes, *et al.*, 1955). Will antibodies which recognize such a channel be useful for identifying inhibitory synapses in the central nervous system? If so, immunocytological studies using such antibodies, which can define inhibitory versus excitatory synapses, in conjunction with neuroanatomical studies may indicate functional pathways. In addition, specific activation of such channels might be mediated by the existence of a second domain on the molecule or linkage of another protein to the channel which serves as a specific receptor for neurotransmitters or neuropeptides.

With the use of monoclonal antibodies it will be possible to identify molecules which encode positional information or "specificity" in the nervous system (see Attardi and Sperry, 1963; Purves *et al.*, 1981; Letinsky *et al.*, 1976). Already, work done by Trisler *et al.* (1981) suggest that this approach is feasible. In chick retina they were able to identify a molecule with use of a monoclonal antibody distributed in a dorsal-ventral gradient. Whether this molecule encodes information for retinotectal specificity is not yet known, but the approach certainly appears promising. Monoclonal antibodies may also be useful to define components in extracellular matrix which influence axons to reinnervate and elaborate synaptic specializations at their original synaptic sites (Marshall *et al.*, 1977; Sanes *et al.*, 1978). These reagents would permit identification of the various components which make up the basal lamina and, if they block the reinnervation process, make it possible to dissect the components responsible for specific reinnervation and perhaps innervation during embryonic development.

Finally, given the complexity of the central nervous system, the importance of obtaining pure cell populations which can be identified and separated with monoclonal antibodies against surface markers for biochemical and physiological analyses cannot be overemphasized (Barnstable, 1980; Zipser and MacKay, 1981). Indeed, an important lesson from studies of immune function is that even small numbers of contaminating cells in a "purified" population can give rise to spurious biochemical and functional data. Whether it will be possible to obtain pure populations of neurons from the central nervous system through clonal expansion is not clear. However, Sieber-Blum and Cohen (1980) have already begun to use clones of neural crest cells to study neuronal lineage and differentiation. With the use of purified and perhaps cloned cell populations, it will be possible to define factors important for survival, growth, and differentiation of individual cell sets and then to examine how these various cell sets establish and maintain functional interactions.

4. REFERENCES

Attardi, D. G., and Sperry, R. W., 1963, Preferential selection of central pathways by regenerating optic fibers, *Exp. Neurol.* **7**:46.

Barnstable, C. J., 1980, Monoclonal antibodies which recognize different cell types in the rat retina, *Nature (London)* **286**:231.

Boyse, E. A., Miyazawa, M., Aoki, T., and Old, L. J., 1968, Ly-A and Ly-B: Two systems of lymphocyte isoantigens in the mouse, *Proc. R. Soc. London Ser. B* **170**:175.

Boyse, E. A., Itakura, K., Stockert, E., Iritani, C. A., and Miura, M., 1971, Ly–C: A third locus specifying alloantigens expressed only on thymocytes and lymphocytes, *Transplantation* **11**:351.

Cantor, H., and Asofsky, R., 1972, Synergy among lymphoid cells mediating the graft-versus-host response. III. Evidence for interaction between two types of thymus-derived cells, *J. Exp. Med.* **135**:764.

Cantor, H., and Boyse, E. A., 1975a, Functional subclasses of T lymphocytes bearing different Ly antigens. I. Generation of functionally distinct T-cell subclasses is a differentiative process independent of antigen, *J. Exp. Med.* **141**:1376.

Cantor, H., and Boyse, E. A., 1975b, Functional subclasses of T lymphocytes bearing different Ly antigens. II. Cooperation between subclasses of Ly$^+$ cells in the generation of killer activity, *J. Exp. Med.* **141**:1390.

Cantor, H., Shen, F. W., and Boyse, E. A., 1976, Separation of helper T cells from suppressor T cells expressing different Ly components. II. Activation by antigen: After immunization, antigen-specific suppressor and helper activities are mediated by distinct T-cell subclasses, *J. Exp. Med.* **143**:1391.

Cantor, H., Hugenberger, J., McVay-Boudreau, L., Eardley, D. D., Kemp, J., Shen, F. W., and Gershon, R. K., 1978, Immunoregulatory circuits among T-cell sets. Identification of a subpopulation of T-helper cells that induces feedback inhibition, *J. Exp. Med.* **148**:871.

Claman, H. N., Chaperon, E. A., and Triplett, R. F., 1966, Thymus-marrow cell combinations. Synergism in antibody production, *Proc. Soc. Exp. Biol. Med.* **122**:1167.

Coombs, J. S., Eccles, J. C., and Fatt, P., 1955, The specific ionic conductances and the ionic movements across the motoneuronal membrane that produce the inhibitory post-synaptic potential, *J. Physiol.* **130**:326.

Dialynas, D. P., Loken, M. R., Glasebrook, A. L., and Fitch, F. W., 1981, Lyt-2$^-$/Lyt-3$^-$ variants of a cloned cytolytic T cell line lack an antigen receptor functional in cytolysis, *J. Exp. Med.* **153**:595.

Durda, P. J., Shapiro, C., and Gottlieb, P. D., 1978, Partial molecular characterization of the Ly-1 alloantigen on mouse thymocytes, *J. Immunol.* **120**:53.

Eardley, D. D., Hugenberger, J., McVay-Boudreau, L., Shen, F. W., Gershon, R. K., and Cantor, H., 1978, Immunoregulatory circuits among T-cell sets. I. T-helper cells induce other T-cell sets to exert feedback inhibition, *J. Exp. Med.* **147**:1106.

Edelman, G. M., 1971, Antibody structure and molecular immunology, *Ann. N.Y. Acad. Sci.* **190**:5.

Finberg, R., Burakoff, S. J., Cantor, H., and Benacerraf, B., 1978, The biologic significance of alloreactivity. II. T cells stimulated by Sendai virus coated syngeneic cells specifically lyse allogeneic target cells, *Proc. Natl. Acad. Sci. U.S.A.* **75:**5145.

Fresno, M., McVay-Boudreau, L., Nabel, G., and Cantor, H., 1981a, Antigen-specific T lymphocyte clones. II. Purification and biological characterization of an antigen-specific suppressive protein synthesized by cloned T cells, *J. Exp. Med.* **153:**1260.

Fresno, M., Nabel, G., McVay-Boudreau, L., Furthmayer, H., and Cantor, H., 1981b, Antigen-specific T lymphocyte clones. I. Characterization of a T lymphocyte clone expressing antigen-specific suppressive activity, *J. Exp. Med.* **153:**1246.

Fresno, M., McVay-Boudreau, L., and Cantor, H., 1982, Antigen-specific T lymphocyte clones. III. Papain splits purified T-suppressor molecules into two functional domains, *J. Exp. Med.,* in press.

Gershon, R. K., 1974, T-cell control of antibody production, *Contemp. Top. Immunobiol* **3:**1.

Glasebrook, A. L., and Fitch, F. W., 1980, Alloreactive cloned T cell lines. I. Interactions between cloned amplifier and cytolytic T cell lines, *J. Exp. Med.* **151:**876.

Hollander, N., Pillemer, E., and Weissman, I. L., 1980, Blocking effect of Lyt-2 antibodies on T cell function, *J. Exp. Med* **152:**674.

Hollander, N., Pillemer, E., and Weissman, I. L., 1981, Effects of Lyt antibodies on T-cell functions: Augmentation by anti-Lyt-1 as opposed to inhibition by anti-Lyt-2, *Proc. Natl. Acad. Sci. U.S.A.* **78:**1148.

Huber, B., Devinsky, O., Gershon, R. K., and Cantor, H., 1976, Cell-mediated immunity: Delayed type hypersensitivity and cytotoxic responses are mediated by different T cell subclasses, *J. Exp. Med.* **143:**1534.

Itakura, K., Hutton, J. J., Boyse, E. A., and Old, L. J., 1972, Genetic linkage relationships of loci specifying differentiation alloantigens in the mouse, *Transplantation* **13:**239.

Jandinski, J., Cantor, H., Tadakuma, T., Peavy, D. L., and Pierce, C. W., 1976, Separation of helper T cells from suppressor T cells expressing different Ly components. I. Polyclonal activation: Suppressor and helper activities are inherent properties of distinct T cell subclasses, *J. Exp. Med.* **143:**1382.

Ledbetter, J. A., and Herzenberg, L. A., 1979, Xenogeneic monoclonal antibodies to mouse lymphoid differentiation antigens, *Immunol Rev.* **47:**63.

Ledbetter, J. A., Seaman, W. E., Tsu, T. T., and Herzenberg, L., 1981, Lyt-2 and Lyt-3 antigens are on two different polypeptide subunits linked by disulfide bonds, *J. Exp. Med.* **153:**1503.

Letinsky, M. S., Fischbeck, K. H., and McMahan, U. J., 1976, Precision of reinnervation of original postsynaptic sites in frog muscle after a nerve crush, *J. Neurophysiol.* **5:**691.

Marshall, L. M., Sanes, J. R., and McMahan, U. J., 1977, Reinnervation of original synaptic sites on muscle fiber membrane after disruption of the muscle cells, *Proc. Natl. Acad. Sci. U.S.A.* **74:**3073.

Miller, J. F. A. P., and Mitchell, G. F., 1968, Immunological activity of thymus and thoracic duct lymphocytes, *Proc. Natl. Acad. Sci. U.S.A.* **59:**296.

Mozes, E., and Haimovich, J., 1979, Antigen-specific T cell helper factor crossreacts idiotypically with antibodies of the same specificity, *Nature (London)* **278:**56.

Murphy, D. B., 1978, The I-J subregion of the murine H-2 gene complex, *Springer Semin. Immunopathol.* **1:**111.

Nabel, G., Fresno, M., Chessman, A., and Cantor, H., 1981, Use of cloned populations of mouse lymphocytes to analyze cellular differentiation, *Cell* **23:**19.

Nakayama, E., Shiku, H., Stockert, E., Oettgen, H. F., and Old, L. J., 1979, Cytotoxic T cells: Lyt phenotype and blocking of killing activity by Lyt antisera, *Proc. Natl. Acad. Sci. U.S.A.* **76:**1977.

Natvig, J. B., and Kunkel, H. G., 1973, Human immunoglobulins: Classes, subclasses, genetic variants, and idiotypes, *Adv. Immunol.* **16**:1.

Purves, D., Thompson, W., and Yip, J. W., 1981, Reinnervation of ganglia transplanted to the neck from different levels of the guinea-pig sympathetic chain, *J. Physiol.* **313**:49.

Reilly, E. B., Auditore-Hargreaves, K., Hämmerling, U., and Gottlieb, P. D., 1980, Lyt-2 and Lyt-3 alloantigens: Precipitation with monoclonal and conventional antibodies and analysis on one- and two-dimensional polyacrylamide gels, *J. Immunol.* **125**:2245.

Sanes, J. R., Marshall, L. M., and McMahan, U. J., 1978, Reinnervation of muscle fiber basal laminar after removal of myofibers. Differentiation of regenerating axons at original synaptic sites, *J. Cell. Biol.* **78**:176.

Sarmiento, M., Glasebrook, A. L., and Fitch, F. W., 1980, IgG or IgM monoclonal antibodies reactive with different determinants on the molecular complex bearing Lyt 2 antigen block T cell-mediated cytolysis in the absence of complement, *J. Immunol.* **125**:2665.

Shen, F. W., Boyse, E. A., and Cantor, H., 1975, Preparation and use of Ly antisera, *Immunogenetics* **2**:591.

Shinohara, N., and Sachs, D. H., 1979, Mouse alloantibodies capable of blocking cytotoxic T-cell function. I. Relationship between the antigen reactive with blocking antibodies and the Lyt 2 locus, *J. Exp. Med.* **150**:432.

Sieber-Blum, M., and Cohen, A. M., 1980, Clonal analysis of quail neural crest cells. They are pluripotent and differentiate *in vitro* in the absence of noncrest cells, *Dev. Biol.* **80**:96.

Takemori, T., and Tada, T., 1975, Properties of antigen-specific suppressive T-cell factor in the regulation of antibody response of the mouse. I. *In vivo* activity and immunochemical characterizations. *J. Exp. Med.* **142**:1241.

Trisler, C. D., Schneider, M. D. and Nirenberg, M., 1981, A topographic gradient of molecules in retina can be used to identify neuron position, *Proc. Natl. Acad. Sci. U.S.A.* **78**:2145.

Zipser, B., and MacKay, R., 1981, Monoclonal antibodies distinguish identifiable neurones in the leech, *Nature (London)* **289**:549.

5

Immunopathologic Disease of the Central Nervous System

MICHAEL B. A. OLDSTONE

1. INTRODUCTION

Several of the chapters in this book are concerned with the definition of antigens specific to the nervous system. Such antigens promise to be of great importance for future investigations in a variety of contexts in cellular neurobiology. An important aspect of neuroimmunology that such studies do not consider is that of the immunopathologic mechanisms operating when these and other antigens in the nervous system provoke an immune response. In the peripheral nervous system, one of the most important examples is that of the response to the acetylcholine receptor underlying experimental and human myasthenic syndromes (see Chapter 1).

Immune-response-mediated injury of the central nervous system (CNS) also can and does occur. It is the intent of this chapter to describe the factors underlying such injury. However, no attempt is made to review all the scientific literature published on immunopathologic injury of the CNS. Rather, concepts drawn from model systems have been selected for the principles they teach, and general concepts of immune response disorders of the CNS are discussed. Finally, the details of selected immunopathologic diseases are presented.

MICHAEL B. A. OLDSTONE   Department of Immunopathology, Scripps Clinic and Research Foundation, La Jolla, Calif. 92037.

2. IMMUNOPATHOLOGIC INJURY OF THE CNS: GENERAL CONCEPTS

Immunologically mediated tissue injury of the CNS basically follows one or both of two pathways. In the first pathway (Fig. 1), components of the immune system react either against specific antigens found uniquely on cells or tissues or against neoantigens, such as viral antigens, expressed on the surfaces of the CNS cells. In the latter instance, immune components react specifically against those antigens that caused their induction or a complex of those antigens with the host histocompatibility antigens in the case of cytotoxic thymus-derived (T) lymphocytes.

The second pathway by which immune reagents cause CNS damage occurs by deposition of antigen–antibody immune complexes. In this instance, antibodies combine with their corresponding antigens in the blood or other body fluids to form complexes that may later become trapped by basement membranes (Figs. 2 and 3), where they cause injury, usually by activating inflammatory mediators (Fig. 4). Such immune complexes not only lodge in glomerular capillaries (Fig. 2) and arteries but also show a predilection for the choroid plexus (Fig. 3), which is composed of tufts of capillaries.

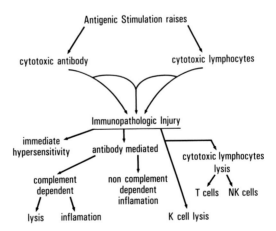

Figure 1. A schematic of various immune reagents involved in immunopathologic injury. T cells: thymus-derived cells; NK cells: natural killer cells; K cell: killer cell [(involved in antibody-dependent cell-mediated killing ADCC)]. See text for discussion of the various immune reactants and their amplifiers.

Immune response *per se* is divided into humoral, cellular, and combined humoral and cellular categories (Fig. 1). The humoral system consists primarily of antibody and complement. Antibody attaches to the antigen that stimulated its production through its Fab'$_2$ binding site. The result is a conformational change of the antibody's Fc portion, readying it for binding to C1, the first component of complement. Thereafter, each component of the complement system is activated sequentially in an autocatalytic manner. For a review of the complement components and both the classical and alternative complement pathways see Müller-Eberhard (1975), Müller-Eberhard and Schreiber (1980), Cooper (1980), and Figs. 4 and 5. Recently, it has become clear that many cells of human origin, including glia and neuronal, when infected with any one of several RNA or DNA viruses, are lysed by specific antiviral antibody and complement, but not by the classical pathway. Instead, cells acutely or persistently infected with and expressing viral antigens on their surfaces are lysed by antiviral antibody and the alternative complement pathway (Fig. 5). In this instance the infected cell itself, in the absence of antibody, activates complement via the alternative pathway (reviewed in Sissons and Oldstone, 1980). Despite the activation of complement components and their binding to the cell surface, lysis does not occur because there is an insufficient buildup of C3b-like molecules on the cell surface. However, upon the addition of specific antiviral antibody, lysis ensues. Antibody by itself cannot lyse virus infected cells, and its activity in conjunction with complement likely functions both by providing more C3b binding sites and by covering membrane bound C3b so as to preclude inactivation by its inactivating enzymes C3b INA and beta 1H (Sissons and Oldstone, 1980).

In the category of cellular immune components are thymus-derived (T) lymphocytes, macrophages, granulocytes, and natural killer (NK) cells. Evidence indicates that recognition of virus-infected cells by cytotoxic T lymphocytes requires not only antigen specificity but also matching of the major histocompatibility complex in the two cell types (reviewed in Zinkernagel and Doherty, 1979). As studied most critically and productively in mice, that portion of the histocompatibility complex associated with cytotoxic T-cell recognition and lysis of virus-infected target cells maps to the D and K region of H-2. Recent evidence indicates that, at least with some virus infections, the lytic process may involve a preference for either the D or the K haplotype. Among the other components of cellular immunity, interest in NK cells has focused on their lack of specificity in killing targets, the possibility that NK cells are a primitive form of T lymphocytes, and their induction and recruitment by interferon (discussed in Welsh, 1978). Cytotoxic lymphocytes (T lymphocytes, NK cells), macrophages, and granulocytes can be attracted to an area of tissue injury via chemotactic factors released by lymphoid cells themselves or by injured target cells. Ordinarily, this process involves cellular release of proteolytic enzymes that cleave nearby complement components, specifically C5, resulting in formation of the C5a chemotactic peptide (Hugli, 1981; Fig. 4).

Humoral and cellular mechanisms may also combine to kill target cells. For example, in antibody-dependent cell-mediated killing (ADCC), specific antibody binds to antigen on the cell surface; then a killer (K) cell binds via the antibody's Fc fragment, the result being lysis of the target cell (reviewed in Perlmann and Cerottini, 1979). Similarly, there are reports of cytophilic macrophages killing cells, presumably by a mechanism that resembles NK-cell-induced injury.

Hence, immunopathologic injury of the CNS can be mediated by the immune system acting directly against unique antigens formed on cells in the nervous system or can be mediated by a secondary reaction of antigen–antibody immune complexes, even those formed at a distant site, and trapped in the vasculature of the CNS. Several disorders of the first type have been reported involving antibodies to neurons, oligodendrocytes, or galactocerebroside, the main component on the surfaces of oligodendrocytes. For example, Williams and his associates (Husby et al., 1976) correlated the appearance and binding of antibodies to neurons in the basal ganglia of patients with chorea to the progress of their disease. Bluestein and his colleagues find that the binding of antibodies to neurons coincides with several of the CNS manifestations seen in patients with systemic lupus erythematosus (Bluestein et al., 1980). Similarly, Silberberg and his associates have shown that the injection of antibody to galactocerebroside causes demyelination (Saida et al., 1979), and the inoculation of myelinated tissues or myelin into animals under the appropriate conditions raises antibodies to galactocerebrosides. In addition to these examples, allergic encephalomyelitis (EAE) is also a model of direct immunologic injury of the nervous system (see below), although the mechanism is largely the result of cytotoxic-T-lymphocyte-mediated injury. These instances of direct-immune-response-mediated tissue damage are one part of the picture. CNS injury also stems from deposition of antigen–antibody immune complexes formed in the body fluids, as exemplified in murine and human systemic lupus (discussed below). To appreciate both pathways of immunopathologically mediated injury, some knowledge of blood flow, immunoglobulin migration, and lymphoid traffic into the CNS is a prerequisite.

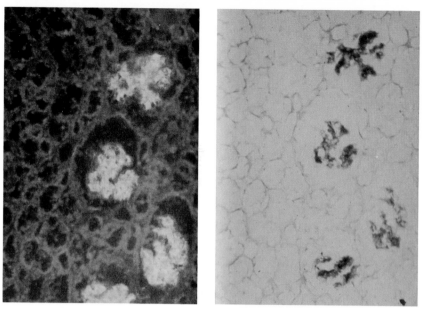

Figure 2. Manifestations of immune complex deposits in the renal glomeruli. Following the injection of ferritin, antibodies to ferritin are elicited and ferritin-antibody to ferritin complexes form in the circulation. Such circulating complexes become deposited in specific sites depending on several factors, including blood flow and the type of endothelial cell and its basement membrane. Left: deposit of host immunoglobulin (antibody to ferritin); right: ferritin in corresponding glomeruli. (Pictures courtesy of Peter Lampert, 1977, *Acta Neuropath.* **38**:83–86.)

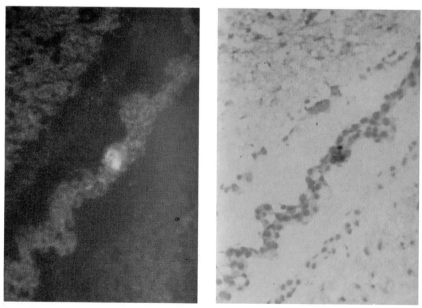

Figure 3. Deposits of ferritin-antibody to ferritin immune complexes in the choroid plexus. From the same section. Left: deposit of host antibody; right: deposit of ferritin. See legend to Fig. 2 and text for details.

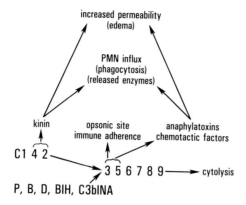

Figure 4. A schematic of the classical (C1, C4, C2) and alternative (P, B, D, B1H, C3bINA) complement pathways and the biological effect of their activated products in immunopathologic injury.

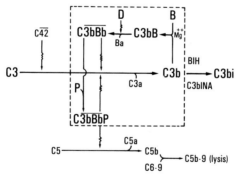

Figure 5. A schematic of the complement pathways with detail of the alternative pathway and the feedback loop. See Müller-Eberhard and Schreiber (1980) and Sissons and Oldstone (1980) for details regarding the complement proteins and their role in lysis of virus-infected cells, respectively. The alternative pathway/amplification system is shown in heavier lettering. By convention major cleavage products of complement proteins are designated b, and minor ones, a; a superscript bar indicates an active enzyme. In this diagram ⤳ indicates a proteolytic cleavage. On the surface of activating particles C3b escapes from regulation and the positive feedback within the enclosed box.

3. BLOOD FLOW AND THE TRAFFIC OF IMMUNOGLOBULIN AND LYMPHOID CELLS IN THE CNS

About 20% of the total body blood flow is delivered to the brain. However, the transport of macromolecules into the CNS is prevented by a barrier composed of astrocytic foot processes bound to the capillary endothelial wall. The concept of this barrier, i.e., blood–brain barrier, dates from Ehrlich's observations (1885) that aniline dyes injected into the bloodstream stained tissues throughout the body but not those of the CNS, with the exception of a few sites within the tuber cinereum, the neurohypophysis, the pineal gland, the spinal ganglia, and the area postrema. However, macromolecules can diffuse into the CNS whenever the blood–brain barrier is altered in permeability owing to injury. Even though macromolecules like immunoglobulin cannot traverse a normal blood–brain barrier, it is believed that lymphoid cells can.

In the presence of a normal blood–brain barrier, antibodies cannot react with the corresponding brain antigens because immunoglobulins cannot diffuse from a vascular component into the CNS parenchyma. This fact embodies two important implications. First, it should not be surprising that experiments involving passive transfers of antibody via the blood stream may not result in CNS disease unless the blood–brain barrier has been injured and becomes permeable. To be meaningful, passive transfers of antibody in the presence of a normal blood–brain barrier require introducing the antibody directly into the ventricular fluids, as evident in several instances. Examples are the reported transfer of experimental allergic encephalitis (J. Simon and O. Simon, 1975; Jankovic et al., 1965) and transfer of the immunopathologic diseases associated with lymphocytic choriomeningitis virus infection (Oldstone and Dixon, 1970) with specific antibodies. The second implication is that the detection of antibodies bound to CNS cells in vivo indicates preceding damage to the blood–brain barrier.

Although immunoglobulin has difficulty penetrating the blood–brain barrier, passively transferred lymphoid cells appear to traverse this impediment readily. Macrophages can enter the blood–brain barrier normally, but it is still unknown whether lymphoblasts do. Some investigators have shown the passage of mononuclear cells across the blood–brain barrier, as pictured in Fig. 6. In several different kinds of experiments with lymphocytes sensitized to brain antigens or to viral antigens, it has been possible to passively transfer lymphoid cells and show their subsequent localization in the CNS (Werdelin and McCluskey, 1971). Using radiolabeled lymphocytes, others have noted that less than 10% of the inflammatory cells in lesions are of donor origin and that target organ specificity is limited, since the radiolabeled donor

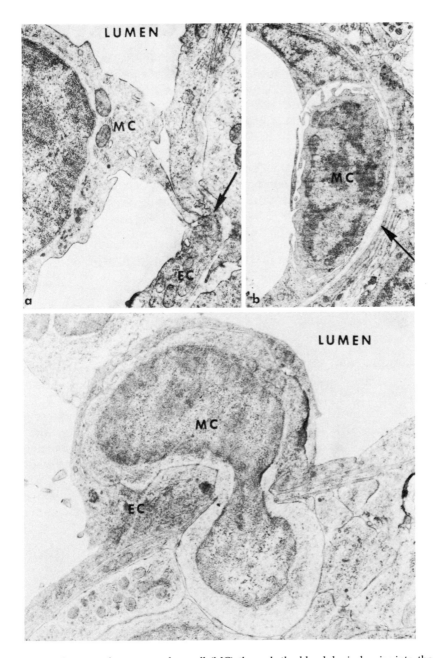

Figure 6. Passage of a mononuclear cell (MC) through the blood–brain barrier into the CNS parenchyma. In panel (a), a pseudopod of the mononuclear cell appears to probe the junction (arrow) of two endothelial cells (EC). In panel (b) the mononuclear cell lies against the basement membrane (arrow). The mononuclear cell is observed passing through the basement membrane and into the brain parenchyma in the panel (c). (Photomicrograph courtesy of Peter Lampert, 1967, *Acta Neuropath.* **9:**99–126.)

lymphoid cells infiltrate to sites other than the CNS. In addition to cytotoxic lymphocytes, it is likely that specifically primed B lymphocytes traverse the blood–brain barrier to enter the CNS. There, they may be confronted with specific antigen, proliferate, differentiate into plasma cells, and release antibody locally in the CNS parenchyma. Support for this concept comes from experiments in which antibody that reacted with myelin basic protein was released by lymphocytes in the CNS parenchyma (Lennon and Carnegie, 1971). Further, there is abundant evidence that antibody is produced within the CNS during the courses of several viral encephalitides and also during diseases like multiple sclerosis (Tourtellotte, 1972; Norrby *et al.*, 1974).

4. MODELS DEPICTING IMMUNOPATHOLOGICALLY MEDIATED INJURY OF THE CNS

4.1. Direct Pathway of Immune Response Injury: Allergic Encephalomyelitis

When encephalitic antigen and adjuvant are injected into the appropriate mammalian host, an autoimmune response and a well-defined disease follow in terms of expected clinical, histopathologic, and immunologic findings (reviewed in Paterson, 1966; Paterson, 1977). CNS tissue, combined with complete Freund's adjuvant, can cause severe acute neurologic disease within 6 to 20 days after inoculation into an autologous, homologous, or heterologous host. The hallmark of allergic encephalomyelitis is focal areas of perivascular lymphocytic infiltration, frequently accompanied by adjacent areas of demyelination (Fig. 7).

It is of interest that historically, both in clinical investigation and in research work, the nervous system is the site where adverse immune

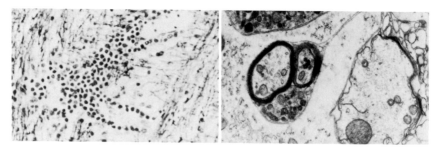

Figure 7. Pathologic events associated with experimental allergic encephalomyelitis. Left: perivascular lymphocyte cuffing; right: accompanying demyelination.

low levels of hemolytically active C4 in these fluids of all 11 patients studied who had clinical findings of CNS lupus. In contrast, C4 was normal in the cerebrospinal fluids of 7 patients with active lupus but without CNS manifestations, 40 patients without neurologic disease, and 50 of 55 patients with various other neurologic disorders. In several patients with active CNS lupus, low levels of C4 hemolytic activity correlated directly with the clinical courses of individual patients. Thus, a patient with active CNS lupus whose C4 hemolytic activity was low became normal in this respect, along with clinical improvement. Other investigators found DNA–anti-DNA antibody complexes in the cerebrospinal fluids of patients with CNS lupus. With my colleague, Peter Lampert, I have studied 4 patients with CNS lupus, and all contained DNA–anti-DNA immune complexes (Fig. 9). One of these 4 patients was studied by Drs. Bluestein and Lampert (see Bluestein *et al.*, 1980) and showed antibody binding to neuronal cells. Other evidence supporting the concept of altered blood–brain barrier permeability accompanying immune complex disease has been presented by Harbeck and his colleagues (1979). These investigators found a direct correlation between deposits of immune complexes in the choroid plexuses of rabbits with acute immune complex disease and an increase in albumin and IgG levels in the animals' cerebrospinal fluids. In addition, complexes containing bovine serum albumin and its antibody were detected in the cerebrospinal fluids of rabbits in which acute immune complex disease was caused by the injection of bovine serum albumin.

5. CONCLUSION

In conclusion, a variety of disorders of the CNS, as well as the peripheral nervous system, are caused by responses of the immune system. This occurs by direct (cytotoxic antibody, lymphocytes) or direct (immune complexes) immune-mediated pathways. Knowledge about the genetic control of immune responses and the functional roles of various lymphocytes and their subsets is increasing. With this information on hand and the ability to manipulate and regulate specific immune responses, the future of understanding and treating these CNS disorders appears promising.

ACKNOWLEDGMENTS

This is Publication No. 2338 from the Department of Immunopathology, Scripps Clinic and Research Foundation, La Jolla, California 92037.

This research was supported by U.S.P.H.S. grants NS-12428, AI-09484, AI-07007, and NS-14068 and by National Multiple Sclerosis Society Research Grant No. 1285-A-4.

6. REFERENCES

Bluestein, H. G., Williams, G. W., and Steinberg, A. D., 1981, Cerebrospinal fluid antibodies to neuronal cells: Association with neuropsychiatric manifestations of systemic lupus erythematosus, *Amer. J. Med.* **70**:241.

Cooper, N. R., 1980, The complement system, in: *Basic and Clinical Immunology*, 3rd ed. (H. H. Fudenberg, D. P. Stites, J. L. Caldwell, and J. V. Wells, eds.), pp. 83–95, Lang Medical Publishers, Palo Alto, Calif.

Erlich, P., 1885, *Das Sauerstaff-Bedürfniss des Organesmus*, August Hiorchwald, Berlin.

Harbeck, R. J., Hoffman, A. A., Hoffman, S. A., and Shucard, D. W., 1979, Cerebrospinal fluid and the choroid plexus during acute immune complex disease. *Clin. Immunol. Immunopathol.* **13**:413.

Hugli, T. E., 1981, The structural basis for anaphylatoxin and chemotactic functions of C3a, C4a, and C5a, *Critical Reviews in Immunology* **1**:321.

Husby, G., Van de Rijn, I., Zabriskie, J. B., Abdin, Z. H., and Williams, Jr., R. C., 1976, Antibodies reacting with cytoplasm of subthalamic and caudate nuclei neurons in chorea and acute rheumatic fever, *J. Exp. Med.* **144**:1094.

Jankovic, B. D., Draskoci, M., and Janjic, M., 1965, Passive transfer of "allergic" encephalomyelitis with antibrain serum injected into the lateral ventricle of the brain, *Nature (London)* **207**:428.

Kabat, E. A., Wolf, A., and Bezer, A. E., 1949, Studies on acute disseminated encephalomyelitis produced experimentally in Rhesus monkeys. IV. Disseminated encephalomyelitis produced in monkeys with their own brain tissue, *J. Exp. Med.* **89**:395.

Lampert, P. W., and Oldstone, M. B. A., 1973, Host IgG and C3 deposits in the choroid plexus during spontaneous immune complex disease, *Science* **180**:408.

Lennon, V. A., and Carnegie, P. R., 1971, Immunopharmacological disease: A break in tolerance to receptor sites, *Lancet* **1**:630.

Morgan, I. M., 1947, Allergic encephalomyelitis in monkeys in response to injection of normal monkey nervous tissue, *J. Exp. Med.* **85**:131.

Müller-Eberhard, H. J., 1975, Complement, *Annu. Rev. Biochem.* **44**:697.

Müller-Eberhard, H. J., and Schreiber, R. D., 1980, Molecular biology and chemistry of the alternative pathway of complement, *Adv. Immunol.* **29**:1.

Norrby, E., Link, H., Olsson, J-E., Panelius, M., Salmi, A., and Vandvik, B., 1974, Comparison of antibodies against different viruses in cerebrospinal fluid and serum samples from patients with multiple sclerosis, *Infect. Immun.* **10**:688.

Oldstone, M. B. A., 1975, Virus neutralization and virus-induced immune complex disease: Virus–antibody union resulting in immunoprotection or immunologic injury—Two different sides of the same coin, in: *Progress in Medical Virology*, Vol. 19 (J. L. Melnick, ed.), pp. 84–119, S. Karger, Basel.

Oldstone, M. B. A., and Dixon, F. J., 1970, Pathogenesis of chronic disease associated with persistent lymphocytic choriomeningitis viral infection. II. Relationship of anti-LCM viral response to tissue injury in chronic disease, *J. Exp. Med.* **131**:1.

Oldstone, M. B. A., and Lampert, P. W., 1974, Immune complex disease in chronic virus infection: Involvement of the choroid plexus, in: *Advances in the Biosciences*, vol. 12 (G. Raspe and S. Bernhard, eds.), pp.. 381–390, Pergamon Press, London.

Ortiz-Ortiz, L., and Weigle, W. O., 1976, Cellular events in the induction of experimental allergic encephalomyelitis in rats, *J. Exp. Med.* **144:**604.

Paterson, P. Y., 1966, Experimental allergic encephalomyelitis and autoimmune diseases, *Adv. Immunol.* **5:**131.

Paterson, P. Y., 1977, Autoimmune neurological disease: Experimental animal systems and implications for multiple sclerosis, in: *Autoimmunity: Genetic, Immunologic, Virologic, and Clinical Aspects* (N. Talal, ed.), pp. 643–692, Academic Press, New York.

Perlmann, P., and Cerottini, J. C., 1979, Cytotoxic lymphocytes, in: *The Antigens*, vol. 5 (M. Sela, ed.), pp. 173–281, Academic Press, New York.

Petz, L. D., Sharp, G. C., Cooper, N. R., and Irvin, W. S., 1971, Serum and cerebral spinal fluid complement and serum autoantibodies in systemic lupus erythematosus, *Medicine* **50:**259.

Rivers, T. M., and Schwentker, F. F., 1935, Encephalomyelitis accompanied by myelin destruction experimentally produced in monkeys, *J. Exp. Med.* **61:**689.

Saida, K., Saida, T., Brown, M. J., and Silberberg, D. H., 1979, *In vivo* demyelination induced by intraneural injection of anti-galactocerebroside serum. A morphologic study, *Am. J. Pathol.* **95:**99.

Simon, J., and Simon, O., 1975, Effect of passive transfer of anti-brain antibodies to a normal recipient, *Exp. Neurol.* **47(3):**523.

Sissons, J. G. P., and Oldstone, M. B. A., 1980, Antibody-mediated destruction of virus-infected cells, *Adv. Immunol.* **29:**209.

Tourtellotte, W. W., 1972, Interaction of local central nervous system immunity and systemic immunity in the spread of multiple sclerosis demyelination, in: *Multiple Sclerosis* (F. Wolfgram, G. W. Ellison, J. G. Stevens, and J. M. Andrews, eds.), p. 285, Academic Press, New York.

Welsh, R. M., Jr., 1978, Mouse natural killer cells: Induction, specificity, and function, *J. Immunol.* **121:**1631.

Werdelin, O., and McCluskey, R. T., 1971, The nature and the specificity of mononuclear cells in experimental autoimmune inflammations and the mechanisms leading to their accumulation, *J. Exp. Med.* **133:**1242.

Zinkernagel, R. M., and Doherty, P. C., 1979, MHC restricted cytotoxic T cells: Studies on the biological role of polymorphic major transplantation antigens determining T cell restriction, specificity, function and responsiveness, *Adv. Immunol.* **27:**52.

6

The Use of Antibodies to Define and Study Major Cell Types in the Central and Peripheral Nervous System

RHONA MIRSKY

1. INTRODUCTION

This chapter outlines research done in the MRC Neuroimmunology Project, Zoology Department, University College London, over the last 10 years. The variety of problems studied is large, but underlying the approach to all of them has been the premise that antibodies can be valuable tools for studying the nervous system.

One of many possible ways to look at how the glia and neurons of the central and peripheral nervous system interact is to use antibodies to define, compare, and isolate subsets of cells. An important goal is to be able to study purified cell populations under controlled conditions, both in isolation and in combination with each other. While this has the severe disadvantage of disturbing the incredibly complex interrelationships of the nervous system observed *in situ*, it has the advantage that some of the molecular mechanisms fundamental to an eventual understanding of these complex interactions can be examined under condi-

RHONA MIRSKY · MRC Neuroimmunology Group, Department of Zoology, University College London, London, England.

141

tions which cannot be achieved in other ways. For example, the interpretation of biochemical measurements of parameters such as protein, DNA, RNA composition, or enzyme levels in subfractions of whole brain or even well-defined brain regions such as cerebellum is complicated by the difficulty of separating out the contributions from the different types of cells. Even in the case of supposedly homogeneous preparations such as synaptosomes the level of contamination from myelin and microsomes is a major problem (Whittaker and Barker, 1972).

Antibodies have been widely used to study the interaction of different cell types in the immune system. By 1971, B and T lymphocytes in mice could be distinguished from one another because B cells expressed immunoglobulin on their surface while T cells possessed the cell surface antigen Thy-1 (Raff, 1970). In the 1970s, functionally distinct subpopulations of B cells could be identified by the different classes of immunoglobulins on their cell surfaces (Parkhouse and Cooper, 1977), while the differential expression of cell surface Lyt antigens enabled different subsets of T cells to be distinguished (Cantor and Boyse, 1977). These and other antigenic markers have been used in conjunction with specific antibodies to study the development, properties, and interactions of an increasing number of functional subclasses of lymphocytes.

In recent years, the development of techniques for making hybridoma cell lines which produce monoclonal antibodies has greatly extended the potential of this approach. In 1975, Köhler and Milstein introduced a method for fusing antibody-secreting B lymphocytes with cultured myeloma cells to produce immortal cell lines, each of which secreted a monoclonal antibody. Since then, monoclonal antibodies have been produced to a large variety of molecules, and in the immune system some of these have been used to clarify the ontogeny and function of T-cell subsets (Ledbetter and Herzenberg, 1979). These antibodies can be used as highly specific probes in a wide variety of biological systems, including the nervous system. Recently, several groups (Eisenbarth et al., 1979; Kennett and Gilbert, 1979; Barnstable, 1980; Lagenaur et al., 1980; Bartlett et al., 1981; Cohen and Selvendran, 1981; Vulliamy et al., 1981) have used these methods to identify antigens unique to subpopulations of the major cell types in both the peripheral (PNS) and central (CNS) nervous system.

2. DEVELOPMENT OF SPECIFIC MARKER SYSTEMS FOR IDENTIFYING THE MAJOR CELL TYPES IN NERVOUS SYSTEM CULTURES

Our earlier work was directed toward the development of antibodies which recognized and differentiated between the major nervous system cell types in culture, and we used a combination of different methods to realize this goal. Whenever practicable, we correlated results obtained in culture with those from frozen sections of nervous tissue. We wished not only to identify cells but also to separate them. Since established immunological methods for cell separation, using positive selection procedures such as the fluorescence-activated cell sorter (FACS) or rosetting, or negative-selection procedures such as antibody and complement-mediated killing, rely on the fact that different cell types express different surface antigens, we concentrated on identifying antibodies which recognize cell surface molecules, although we have also used antibodies to intracellular antigens to define certain cell types.

To characterize the distribution of various antigens on cells within the nervous system, primary cultures of dissociated cells from perinatal and fetal rats were used. By utilizing nervous system cultures from a wide variety of areas from both the peripheral and central nervous system we have been able to screen the major nervous system cell types for the presence or absence of a specified molecule. Cultures from well-defined areas such as sciatic nerve, dorsal root ganglion (DRG), superior cervical ganglion (SCG), nodose ganglion, and myenteric plexus in the peripheral nervous system, and from cerebellum, cerebrum, corpus callosum, optic nerve, retina, and spinal cord from the CNS contain several different cell types and were examined for antibody binding to either surface or intracellular molecules by indirect immunofluorescence.

The major cell types found in or associated with nervous system cultures include neurons, astrocytes, oligodendrocytes, Schwann cells, fibroblasts, leptomeningeal cells, and ependymal cells, as well as phagocytic cells including microglia, and we have defined markers which enable us to distinguish between them.

In many studies we used combinations of antibodies raised in different species such as mouse or rabbit together with second antibodies conjugated to either tetramethyl rhodamine or fluorescein to detect whether the two antigens are present on the same, overlapping, or completely separate cell populations.

Table I summarizes the results which will now be described in detail in the text.

2.1. Rat Neural Antigen-1: A Rat Schwann-Cell-Specific Surface Antigen

Initially it seemed that one of the best ways to raise antibodies which would recognize surface molecules on specific cell types in the nervous system would be to immunize mice and rabbits with tumor cell lines of defined origin, such as neuroblastomas, astrocytomas, oligodendrogliomas, and Schwannomas. A large number of tumor cell lines

Table I. Cell Type Distribution of Major Markers in Nervous System Cultures

Marker	Neurons		Schwann cells	Enteric glia	Astrocytes	Oligodendrocytes	Fibroblasts	Leptomeningeal cells	Ependymal cells	Macrophages	Positive species
	CNS	PNS									
Tetanus toxin	+	+	−	−	+/−[a]	−	−	−	−	−	Vertebrates
Ran-1	−	−	+	+	−	−	−	−	−	−	Rat
Thy-1	+/−[b]	+	−	−	+/−[c]	−	−	+/−[d]	−	−	Human[e], rat, mouse
Fibronectin	−	−	−	−	−	−	+	+	−	−	Human, rat, mouse, guinea pig, chick
GFAP	−	−	+/−[f]	+	+	−	−	−	−	−	Human, rat, mouse, guinea pig (weak), chick[g]
GalC	−	−	+/−[h]	−	−	+	−	−	−	−	Vertebrates
Ran-2	−	−	−	−	+	−	−	+	+	−	Rat
A4	+	−	−	−	+/−	−	−	−	−	−	Human, sheep, rabbit, rat, bovine, pig
38/D7	−	+	−	−	−	−	−	−	−	−	Rat
Phagocytosis	−	−	−	−	−	−	−	−	−	+	—
Fc receptor	−	−	−	−	−	−	−	−	−	+	—
Cilia	−	−	−	−	−	−	−	−	+	−	—

[a] Fibrous astrocytes in optic nerve cultures bind both tetanus toxin and monoclonal antibody A4 weakly.
[b] Present on some but not all neurons in culture.
[c] Present on some astrocytes from newborn rat after 1 week in culture.
[d] Present on a small proportion of leptomeningeal cells.
[e] Antibody to human Thy-1 must be used.
[f] Schwann cells in newborn cultures are GFAP−, but in adult nerve and cultures from 11-day sciatic nerve a few Schwann cells are GFAP+.
[g] Antibody to chick GFAP must be used.
[h] Schwann cells are negative after 3 days in culture, but some are GalC+ on first plating.

of defined origin were induced in inbred rats with the carcinogen ethyl-nitrosourea (ENU). When injected into perinatal rats, ENU induces tumors of the peripheral and central nervous system in a majority of animals. Many *in vitro* cell lines from these tumors were established and subsequently used for injection. Other laboratories, using this general strategy, have had some success (Schachner *et al.*, 1976; Akeson and Seeger, 1977; Stallcup and Coles, 1976), and a dozen or more surface antigens present on neural tumors and usually shared by some cell types in normal brain have been described.

However, in this group, the results were, with one exception, very disappointing. The antibodies raised in this way all reacted with a variety of neural and nonneural tissues. Only one recognized an antigen present on a single cell type in the nervous system.

This antiserum, raised in C3H mice against a cell line 33B derived from a tumor arising in the spinal cord and adjacent nerve roots, proved interesting. After extensive absorption with rat spleen, thymus, liver, and fibroblasts the antiserum reacted with a cell surface antigen named rat neural antigen-1 (Ran-1). It was shared by all rat neural tumors tested, including gliomas, Schwannomas, and neuroblastomas, but was absent on a variety of nonneural tumors. By adsorption assays the antigen was most abundant in adult peripheral nerve and fetal tissue, but was also detectable in adult brain and in kidney (Fields *et al.*, 1975).

To determine which cell types in the nervous system expressed the Ran-1 antigen, its distribution was first examined in primary dissociated cell cultures of newborn sciatic nerve (Brockes *et al.*, 1977). These cultures contain only fibroblasts and Schwann cells, and it was known already (Stern, 1973) that fibroblasts could be identified by the Thy-1 antigen expressed on their cell surface. This antigen was originally defined as being present on thymocytes, brain, and nerves (Reif and Allen, 1964), but it has subsequently been found on a variety of cell types.

Incubation of sciatic nerve cultures with mouse anti-Ran-1 together with rabbit anti-Thy-1.1 followed by tetramethyl-rhodamine-conjugated goat anti-mouse immunoglobulin (goat anti-MIgRd) and fluorescein-conjugated goat anti-rabbit Ig (goat anti-RIgRd) revealed that the Ran-1 and Thy-1 antigens were each present on about 50% of the cells in the culture and that the distribution of the antigens was mutually exclusive. This indicated that Ran-1 was expressed only by Schwann cells in these cultures, while Thy-1 was expressed only by fibroblasts (Brockes *et al.*, 1977) (Fig. 1). Furthermore, in cultures from newborn DRG and SCG which contain neurons in addition to Schwann cells and fibroblasts, only the Schwann cells expressed the Ran-1 antigen (Fields *et al.*, 1978).

In most cultures from optic nerve, cerebellum, corpus callosum,

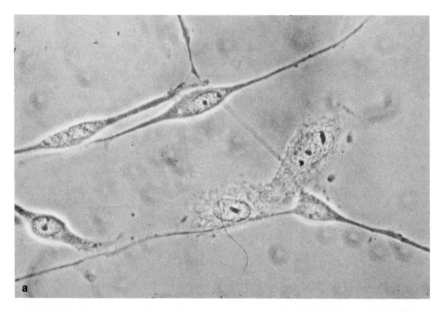

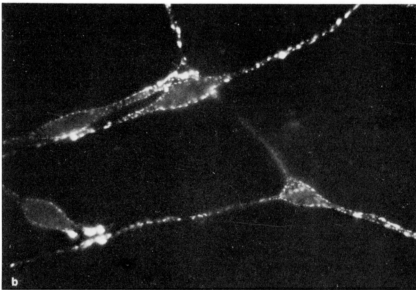

Figure 1. Ran-1$^+$ Schwann cell. Cultures of newborn rat sciatic nerve were incubated for 30 min at room temperature with mouse anti-Ran-1, followed by goat anti-MIgRd and viewed with phase contrast (a) and fluorescence (b) optics. Note the two flat unlabeled fibroblastic cells in the background.

and meninges there were small numbers (<1%) of Ran-1$^+$ cells which had a characteristic (usually bipolar) morphology somewhat resembling Schwann cells seen in sciatic nerve or DRG cultures. In confluent cultures they were often seen on top of a monolayer of flat cells. The Ran-1$^+$ cells were not labeled with any of the other cell-type-specific antisera to be described later in this article, so they are unlikely to be neurons, astrocytes, or oligodendrocytes (Raff *et al.*, 1979).

Interestingly, the glial cells of the enteric plexuses, which have sometimes been classified as Schwann or satellite cells because they are derived from the neural crest (Cook and Burnstock, 1976) but which ultrastructurally and immunohistochemically resemble astrocytes (Gabella, 1972; Jessen and Mirsky, 1980) (see Section 2.3), also express Ran-1 (K.R. Jessen and R. Mirsky, unpublished observations).

The presence of Ran-1 on all rat neural tumors tested (Fields *et al.*, 1975) indicates that cell lines cannot always be used as reliable predictors of the surface properties of the primary cell type from which they are derived.

To identify the major types of nervous system cells other than Schwann cells in culture we used a combination of different antisera, all of which were made by us or by others by immunizing either rabbits or mice with proteins or glycolipids suspected or known to be made by a particular cell type. Although several of the antisera had been used previously to characterize individual cell types *in situ* or in culture, their use in combination with each other enabled us to determine which antigens were confined to a particular cell type, which ones were shared and under what circumstances, and also allowed an estimate of the proportion of different cell types in cultures from various areas of the nervous system.

2.2. Tetanus Toxin: A Cell Surface Marker for Neuronal Cells in Culture

Tetanus toxin, a protein of mol. wt. 150,000 secreted by the bacterium *Clostridium tetanii*, is one of the most potent neurotoxins known. It binds specifically and with high affinity to the surface of neurons and thus affords a means of identifying them in culture. The toxin binds to the gangliosides G_{T1} and G_{D1b} (Van Heyningen, 1963). In 1977 Dimpfel *et al.* showed that ^{125}I tetanus toxin attached only to cells with neuronal morphology in cultures from newborn mouse spinal cord and brain. Later, we used tetanus toxin in conjunction with toxin specific antibodies and indirect immunofluorescence to extend this observation. We showed that the toxin could be used as a specific marker to identify neurons in cultures from the PNS and CNS of rat and chick (Mirsky *et al.*, 1978) (Fig. 2). The great majority of neurons in all cultures so far examined bind the toxin while nonneuronal cells, including most astrocytes, oligodendrocytes, Schwann cells and fibroblasts, are unlabeled. Fibrous astrocytes in newborn optic nerve cultures which contain glial fibrillary acidic protein (GFAP) are an unexplained exception since they bind the toxin weakly (Raff *et al.*, 1979). Human fetal DRG neurons (Kennedy *et al.*, 1980) and amphibian neurons also bind toxin (Vulliamy and Messenger, 1981). Problems sometimes encountered with nonspecific binding of toxin to nonneuronal cells can be minimized by the use of purified tetanus toxin and F(ab')₂ fragments of toxin antibodies if rabbit antitoxin is used. Despite the obvious dangers of using a molecule as potentially lethal as tetanus toxin, it has the advantage that users are readily immunized and antiserum to tetanus toxoid is easily made in rabbits, horses, humans, and mice.

2.3. Glial Fibrillary Acidic Protein: An Intracellular Marker for Astrocytes and Enteric Glial Cells

Glial fibrillary acid protein (GFAP), a cytoskeletal intracellular protein, was originally isolated from human brain (Eng *et al.*, 1971). It is a protein of subunit molecular mass 49–50,000 daltons. A series of stud-

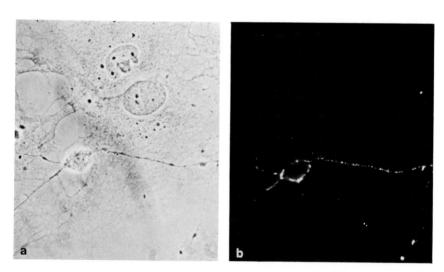

Figure 2. Tetanus toxin⁺ neuron. Cells in cultures of newborn rat cerebral cortex were labeled after 5 days with tetanus toxin, then F(ab')₂ rabbit anti-tetanus toxin, followed by goat anti-RIgRd and viewed with phase contrast (a) and rhodamine (b) optics. Note that only the neuron is labeled.

ies using frozen tissue sections from brain in a variety of species combined with the use of antibodies to GFAP and immunfluorescence and immunoperoxidase techniques established that in the CNS, GFAP is associated with the 10-nm glial intermediate filaments found only in astrocytes or associated cells such as the Bergmann glia of the cerebellum (Bignami *et al.*, 1972; Bignami and Dahl, 1973, 1974; Schachner *et al.*, 1977). It had also been localized in astrocytes in primary tissue culture explants from human fetal CNS (Antanitus *et al.*, 1975), and in newborn rat brain cultures (Bock *et al.*, 1977). To determine its specificity for astrocytes in rat nervous system cultures we used it in combination with the other markers which we developed for the identification of cell types in culture using double-fluorochrome immunofluorescence (see Table I). In contrast to the cell surface antigens, intracellular GFAP can only be visualized by indirect immunofluorescence after permeabilizing the cells (for example, by fixing them for 10 min with 95% ethanol/5% acetic acid) and shows a highly characteristic fibrillar staining pattern (Fig. 3).

GFAP$^+$ cells in the cultures are of two distinct morphological types. The first have a flat, fibroblastic appearance with large, pale nuclei and abundant cytoplasm; the second have processes, often extended and branched, and are smaller and darker than the first type of cell. These may correspond to the protoplasmic and fibrous astrocytes found *in situ*. GFAP$^+$ cells are abundant in 1-week cultures from 5- to 6-day optic nerve, newborn to 8-day cerebellum, newborn cerebral cortex, and 5- to 6-day corpus callosum, are infrequent in cultures of meninges, and are absent in newborn sciatic nerve or DRG cultures. In cerebellum and cerebral cortex cultures more than 90% of GFAP$^+$ cells have fibroblastic morphology, while in corpus callosum or optic nerve cultures half or more of the GFAP$^+$ cells are process-bearing, which is consistent with the distribution of protoplasmic and fibrous astrocytes *in vivo* (Raff *et al.*, 1979).

With two exceptions, GFAP$^+$ astrocytes are negative for the other cell-type-specific markers used to distinguish between cells. The first exception, the presence of GFAP$^+$, tetanus toxin$^+$ process-bearing astrocytes in optic nerve cultures, has already been mentioned. The second exception is the presence of GFAP$^+$, Thy-1.1$^+$ astrocytes in cerebellum and corpus callosum cultures from 5- to 6-day rats kept in culture for more than 1 week. After 16 days in culture about half the astrocytes are Thy-1$^+$, and in cultures of corpus callosum and cerebellum from a 7-month rat again between 30 and 60% of the astrocytes are Thy-1$^+$ 9 days after plating (Pruss, 1979). Astrocytes in both the fibroblastic and process-bearing morphological categories are Thy-1$^+$.

Until recently GFAP had not been found associated with glial cells

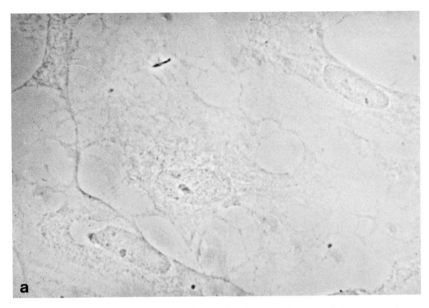

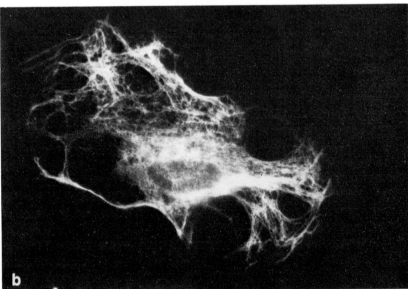

Figure 3. GFAP$^+$, Ran-2$^+$ astrocyte. Cells in cultures of 5-day rat corpus callosum were labeled with mouse anti-Ran-2 antibodies, followed by goat anti-MIgRd, fixed, then labeled with rabbit anti-GFAP and fluorescein-conjugated goat anti-rabbit Ig (goat anti-RIgFl) and viewed with phase contrast (a), fluorescein (b), and rhodamine (c) optics.

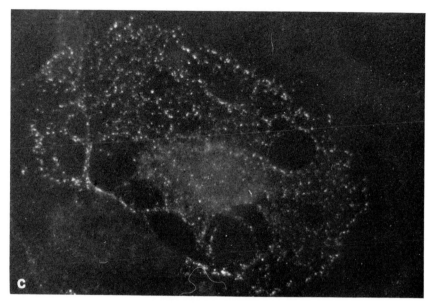

Figure 3 (*continued*).

in the PNS. GFAP$^+$ cells are not found in cultures from newborn or 5- to 6-day rat sciatic nerve or DRG, suggesting that Schwann cells do not normally express GFAP. However, recent experiments (Yen and Fields, 1981) suggest that in adult sciatic nerve a minority of Schwann cells show GFAP-like immunoreactivity, so that there may be some conditions under which Schwann cells can express this antigen. Also, in cultures from 11-day rat sciatic nerve a minority of Schwann cells stain with anti-GFAP sera (R. Mirsky, unpublished observations).

In 1980, Jessen and Mirsky found both in frozen sections and in tissue culture that when cells of the myenteric and submucous plexuses in the gut are treated with anti-GFAP antisera, the glial cells stain in a filamentous pattern highly reminiscent of that seen in GFAP$^+$ astrocytes. Frozen tissue sections from SCG and DRG show no such immunoreactivity. As mentioned in a previous section, the enteric glial cells possess several ultrastructural characteristics in common with astrocytes despite the fact that they are derived from the neural crest.

2.4. Galactocerebroside: A Cell Surface Marker for Oligodendrocytes in Culture

Oligodendrocytes in the CNS and Schwann cells in the PNS both make myelin sheaths which surround the larger nerves and facilitate conduction of the nerve impulse. The major glycolipid in myelin is galactocerebroside (GalC). Sternberger *et al.* (1978*a,b*) using the PAP technique on fixed frozen sections of rat brain, showed that myelin sheaths could be visualized with antiserum to GalC, but they were unable to detect labeling associated with the surface membrane of the oligodendrocytes. Using immunofluorescence, we showed subsequently that GalC is present on the cell surface of oligodendrocytes in cultures of 6-day rat optic nerve which are devoid of neurons (Fig. 4) (Raff *et al.*, 1978*a*). This implies that oligodendrocytes do not require the presence of neurons for the expression of galactocerebroside. GFAP$^+$, tetanus toxin$^+$, and Thy-1$^+$ cells in cultures from optic nerve, corpus callosum, cerebellum, and cerebral cortex do not label with GalC antiserum, while GalC$^+$ cells are negative for GFAP, Thy-1, fibronectin, and Ran-1 and do not bind tetanus toxin, indicating that GalC expression is confined to oligodendrocytes (Raff *et al.*, 1979). GalC$^+$ oligodendrocytes make up about 5% of the cells in cultures of optic nerve and corpus callosum and a somewhat lower percentage in cerebellum and cerebral cortex cultures. They almost all have long, extensively branched processes, and some end in large, membranous expansions (Fig. 4) clearly visible by immunofluorescence but difficult to see by phase contrast microscopy.

In sciatic nerve, DRG, or SCG cultures plated for more than 3 days, Schwann cells do not normally make immunohistochemically detectable amounts of GalC. In very early cultures under some conditions (see Section 4.2), Schwann cells expressing GalC on their surface can be detected.

2.5. Identification of Other Major Cell Types, Including Fibroblasts, Leptomeningeal Cells, and Macrophages

Fibroblasts can be identified in culture by the expression of two surface antigens. The first, Thy-1, has already been mentioned in Section 2.1. However, since some neurons (Mirsky and Thompson, 1975; Currie *et al.*, 1977; Fields *et al.*, 1978) and astrocytes (Pruss, 1979) in culture can also express this antigen, antiserum to fibronectin (LETS) can be used in conjunction with anti-Thy-1 to confirm the identity of fibroblasts in nervous system cultures. Fibronectin is a large protein of molecular mass 210,000 daltons which is made by fibroblasts (Hynes, 1973; Wartiovaara, 1974) and enhances cell adherence. Fibroblasts are generally Thy-1$^+$ and fibronectin$^+$ and do not stain with antisera to GFAP, GalC, tetanus toxin, or Ran-1.

In leptomeningeal and optic nerve cultures many of the flat fibroblastic looking cells are Thy-1$^-$ and GFAP$^-$. In double-labeling exper-

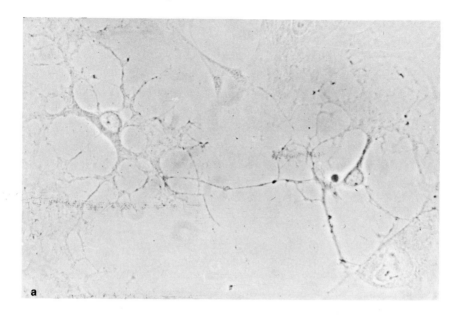

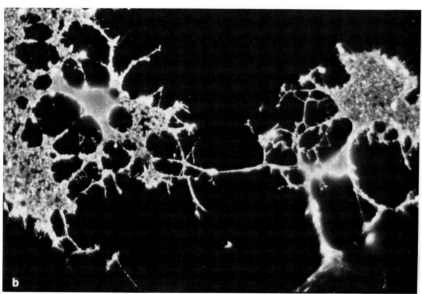

Figure 4. GalC$^+$ oligodendrocytes. Cells in cultures of 5-day rat cerebellum were labeled after 6 days with rabbit anti-GalC followed by goat anti-RIgRd and viewed with phase contrast (a) and fluorescence (b) optics. Note that only the two oligodendrocytes are labeled and that some of their processes end in large, membranous expansions.

iments with anti-GFAP these cells do not label with anti-GalC, anti-Ran-1 or tetanus toxin. However, a majority of them stain in a characteristic extracellular pattern with antifibronectin serum. In leptomeningeal cultures more than 90% of cells have fibroblastic morphology and most of these are fibronectin$^+$ Thy-1$^-$. This suggests that many though not all leptomeningeal cells can be distinguished antigenically from fibroblasts because many of them are fibronectin$^+$ Thy-1$^-$, while fibroblasts are fibronectin$^+$, Thy-1$^+$ (Raff et al., 1979) (see Section 3.3 for a further discussion of this point).

In our cultures GFAP$^+$ astrocytes never express fibronectin; neither do neurons, nor oligodendrocytes, nor Schwann cells. In an immunoperoxidase study of fibronectin distribution in frozen sections of whole rat brain Schachner et al. (1978) found that only fibroblasts, endothelial cells, choroid epithelial cells, and leptomeningeal cells have fibronectin associated with them, while other cell types do not.

Macrophages, presumably including microglia, can be identified in neural cultures by two characteristic properties (Raff et al., 1979). When exposed to latex particles for 1 hr at 37°C, they ingest large numbers of the particles. Occasionally GalC$^+$ oligodendrocytes have latex particles associated with their processes or cell bodies, but no other cell type in either PNS or CNS cultures has latex associated with it. The macrophages also bind and ingest fluorescent conjugates of intact IgG molecules (e.g., goat anti-RIgFl), but not F(ab')$_2$ fragments of these conjugates (Fig. 5). When cells are incubated at 4°C with fluorescent IgG in the presence of sodium azide to inhibit endocytosis, the macrophages show surface labeling. By using F(ab')$_2$ fragments of Ran-1, tetanus toxin, and GalC antibodies, macrophages can be shown to be Ran-1$^-$, GalC$^-$, and not to express receptors for tetanus toxin.

A major cell type not defined by any of the marker molecules described so far is ependymal cells, most of which can be recognized in suspension and in culture by their beating cilia. A monoclonal antibody which recognizes an antigen (Ran-2) present on the surface of astrocytes, ependymal cells, Müller cells, and leptomeningeal cells (Bartlett et al., 1981) will be described in Section 3.6.

3. MONOCLONAL ANTIBODIES

3.1. Introduction

The advantages offered by monoclonal antibodies over conventional heteroantisera in characterizing different cell subpopulations within the nervous system can be exploited in two ways. By making monoclonal

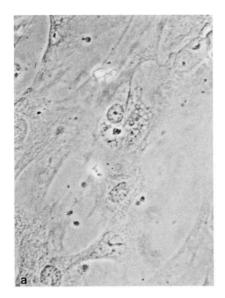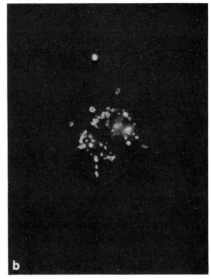

Figure 5. Fc-receptor labeling of microglial cells. Cells in cultures of 5-day rat cerebellum were labeled after 6 days with goat anti-RIgRd and viewed with phase contrast (a) and fluorescence (b) optics. Note the vesicular pattern of staining in (b).

antibodies to well-characterized molecules known to be specific to sub-populations of cells within the nervous system it is possible to produce a range of immunochemical reagents comparable in ease of use to some of the established histochemical techniques. Furthermore, the versatility of the method is potentially greater since few of the older techniques have been able to distinguish subclasses of the major cell types.

An example of this approach is the monoclonal antibody to sub-stance P made by Cuello *et al.* (1979). It is likely that monoclonal anti-bodies to a wide range of peptide neurotransmitters and transmitter specific enzymes such as choline acetyltransferase will soon be available. Since monoclonal antibodies directed against different antigenic sites within the same molecule can be derived, it should be possible to dissect out the contributions which the various domains of the molecule make to the physiological role of that molecule. In addition there is the ines-timable advantage of having a limitless supply of an antibody of defined specificity.

One of the monoclonal antibodies raised in this laboratory against human GFAP falls into this category and will be described in detail in Section 3.2.

Another way of using monoclonal antibodies to define subpopu-lations of the major cell types within the nervous system is to use a method which has been successfully exploited by immunologists, especially in the characterization of surface antigens. Instead of using a single molecule or small group of molecules as immunogen, whole cells (for example, DRG neurons), which contain thousands of potentially immunogenic molecules, are used. By making the screening of antibody-producing clones highly selective, only those hybridomas secreting monoclonal antibodies which distinguish antigens specific to distinct populations of cells (either by their surface characteristics or intracellularly) are chosen for cloning and characterization.

Three monoclonal antibodies produced in this way have been raised in this laboratory and will be further described in subsequent subsections. The first recognizes an antigen present on the surface of astrocytes, ependymal cells, Müller cells, and leptomeningeal cells, the second recognizes an antigen restricted to the surface of neurons in the rat CNS, while the third recognizes an antigen present on the surface of rat peripheral neurons.

3.2. A Monoclonal Antibody to a Common Intermediate-Filament Antigen

Using well-characterized molecules as immunogens for the production of monoclonal antibodies can sometimes yield surprising results. Recently, a hybridoma producing monoclonal antibodies directed against an antigenic determinant on the GFAP molecule was made (Pruss et al., 1981). C3H/He mice were immunized with a partially purified preparation of GFAP prepared from human postmortem spinal cord by the method of Dahl and Bignami (1976). Using polyethylene glycol, spleen cells from these mice were fused with the non-Ig-secreting myeloma P3/NS1/1-Ag4-1 by the method of Galfre et al. (1977). A stable cell line making monoclonal antibodies which recognized an antigenic determinant on GFAP was cloned twice by limiting dilution on layers of peritoneal macrophages as described elsewhere (Bartlett et al., 1981). Using double-fluorochrome immunofluorescence with rabbit anti-GFAP antibodies and radioimmunoassays on acid/alcohol-fixed primary dissociated cell cultures from 5- to 6-day old rat corpus callosum, it was established that the antibody binds to glial filaments present in astrocytes in these cultures. It also binds to filaments in astrocytes in cerebellar, cerebrum, and optic nerve cultures.

Further screening of both PNS and CNS cultures reveals that the monoclonal antibody labels intermediate filaments present in most of the cells examined, including astrocytes, neurons, Schwann cells, and fibroblasts. However, convincing labeling of the neurons usually requires prior fixation with paraformaldehyde and alcohol, which eliminates binding to other cell types. The antibody also binds to myoblasts and myotubes in primary muscle cultures as well as the Z lines in frozen sections of skeletal and cardiac muscle. Colchicine treatment of astrocytes and 3T3 fibroblasts results in the formation of perinuclear coils, a behavior typical of most intermediate-filament types. In PtK2 cells, which contain both vimentin and cytokeratin filaments, colchicine treatment results in the collapse of both the vimentin filaments and the cytokeratin filaments (Osborn et al., 1980), and both filament types can be visualized with antibody to intermediate-filament antigen (anti-IFA).

To confirm that the monoclonal antibody binds to all classes of intermediate filaments an extensive series of protein and filament preparations was analysed by a combination of SDS polyacrylamide gel electrophoresis and immunoautoradiography (Burridge, 1978). In proteins prepared from bovine brain, and from rat brain and spinal cord, the antibody reacts with all three components of the neurofilament triplet (Hoffman and Lasek, 1975) with GFAP and also vimentin. An additional 66,000-dalton polypeptide is also labeled in these and all other preparations tested. The two neurofilament proteins of *Myxicola infundibulum* and squid axoplasm (Gilbert et al., 1975; Roslansky et al., 1980) and the 66,000-dalton polypeptide also label with antibody. Keratins in PtK2 cells and extracted from bovine hoof are also recognized by the antibody, as are purified preparations of both vimentin and desmin.

Thus, this antibody binds to the protein of all five of the major classes of intermediate filaments, indicating that these proteins share a common or closely related antigenic domain which has been highly conserved in evolution and which is therefore almost certainly of functional importance. This determinant is unlike the determinants recognized by conventional heteroantisera to different types of intermediate filaments, which recognize antigenic domains specific to neurofilaments, GFAP, vimentin, desmin, or tonofilaments (Lazarides, 1980). This determinant thus provides the first direct evidence for homology between the different intermediate filaments, although this homology has been suggested previously on the basis of structural studies (Steinert et al., 1980) that intermediate filaments, by analogy with antibodies (Lazarides, 1980), might be constructed from regions of constant and variable size.

In addition, the 66,000-dalton protein with which the antibody reacts is present in all cells and cytoskeletal preparations examined. It stains only weakly with Coomassie blue dye but labels heavily with antibody. It thus resembles the 68,000-dalton protein recently described by Wang et al. (1980) which is associated with intermediate filaments in a variety of nonneuronal and neuronal cells and with myofibril Z lines. While our findings support their suggestion that this protein is a common subunit of various classes of intermediate filaments, they do not support the suggestion that it is identical with the smallest neurofilament protein, since it can be clearly separated from it by its higher mobility in SDS gels. We have suggested that this protein is a subunit shared by all intermediate filaments (Pruss *et al.*, 1981).

3.3. Rat Neural Antigen-2: A Cell Surface Antigen Common to Astrocytes, Ependymal Cells, Müller Cells, and Leptomeninges Defined by a Monoclonal Antibody

Since GFAP is an intracellular protein and therefore cannot be used to identify or purify living astrocytes in culture, it was thought that a monoclonal antibody which would recognize astrocyte-specific surface antigens would be useful. Therefore, as a first step toward this goal Bartlett *et al.* (1981) made a monoclonal antibody which recognized an antigen on the cell surface of astrocytes, ependymal cells, Müller cells, and leptomeningeal cells.

BALB/c mice were immunized three times with cells from cultures of cerebellum from 5- to 6-day rats, devoid of neurons and enriched for astrocytes by treatment with anti-Thy 1 and complement to eliminate fibroblasts (Brockes *et al.*, 1979). Spleen cells from immunized mice were fused with the myeloma P3/NS1/1-Ag4-1 and a stable line-secreting monoclonal antibody named anti-Ran-2$^-$ was isolated after cloning twice by limiting dilution. By radioimmunoassay on astrocyte cultures and T cells the antibody showed high binding to astrocytes and low binding to thymocytes.

The antibody's cell-type distribution was determined by double-fluorochrome immunofluorescence experiments. In rat cerebellum and corpus callosum cultures 90–98% of the GFAP$^+$ cells show labeling of varying intensity with Ran-2 antibodies (Fig. 3). Most of the Ran-2$^-$, GFAP$^+$ cells have the morphology of fibrous astrocytes, and since the variation in staining intensity for Ran-2 between cells is quite large, these probably represented one end of a continuum. Tetanus toxin$^+$ neurons and GalC$^+$ oligodendrocytes are all Ran-2$^-$. A few cells are Ran-2$^+$, GFAP$^-$.

In retinal cultures there are two major cell types: (1) tetanus toxin$^+$ neurons and (2) flat GFAP$^-$, Thy 1$^-$, fibronectin$^-$, Ran-1$^-$ cells which are almost certainly Müller cells. These cells are all Ran-2$^+$ by immunofluorescence.

In cultures of meninges 90% of the cells are Ran-2$^+$, and only about 5% of these are GFAP$^+$. More than 90% of the Ran-2$^+$ cells are also fibronectin$^+$, and of these about 5–10% are also Thy 1$^+$. Since most leptomeningeal cells have been characterized previously as fibronectin$^+$, Thy 1$^-$ (Raff *et al.*, 1979), it was concluded that although most leptomeningeal cells are Ran-2$^+$, Thy 1$^-$, fibronectin$^+$, a minority are Ran-2$^+$, Thy 1$^+$, fibronectin$^+$, and this may possibly reflect a difference between pia and arachnoid cells. Since fibroblasts in sciatic nerve and muscle cultures are Ran-2$^-$, the Ran-2$^+$, Thy 1$^+$, fibronectin$^+$ cells in leptomeningeal cultures are unlikely to be fibroblasts.

Eighty-five to 95% of ciliated ependymal cells in suspensions from dissociated 5- to 6-day rat cerebrum are Ran-2$^+$, and ciliated ependymal cells prepared from neonatal corpus callosum cultures kept *in vitro* for 4–8 weeks are all Ran-2$^+$. Ependymal cells are unlabeled by tetanus toxin or antibodies to GFAP, GalC, Ran-1, Thy 1, or fibronectin (Bartlett *et al.*, 1981).

In cultures of the developing rat nervous system made by dissociation of 10-day embryo brain, Ran-2 is expressed on some flat cells after 1 day in culture. Some of these cells start to make immunohistochemically detectable amounts of GFAP after 5–6 days in culture (Abney *et al.*, 1981) (see Section 4.3), so that some of the Ran-2$^+$, GFAP$^-$ cells seen in cerebellum and corpus callosum cultures are probably astrocyte precursors.

It is perhaps unsurprising that astrocytes, Müller cells, and ependymal cells, all thought to derive from a common precursor cell in the neural tube (Fleischhauer, 1972), should express a common surface antigen. The presence of Ran-2 on leptomeningeal cells is more surprising and is at present unexplained. The embryological origin of leptomeningeal cells is uncertain. Though some experiments have suggested they may derive from the neural crest, other experiments suggest a mesodermal or mixed origin (Shantha and Bourne, 1968). In any case, their origin is clearly different from that of astrocytes, ependymal cells, or Müller cells.

3.4. Neuronal Cell Surface Antigens in the CNS and PNS Recognized by Monoclonal Antibodies

Our first attempt to make monoclonal antibodies which would recognize surface antigens specific to subclasses of neurons in either the CNS or PNS yielded interesting results. Both of the antibodies raised in this laboratory against neurons identified surface antigens which distinguished central neurons from peripheral neurons. This result

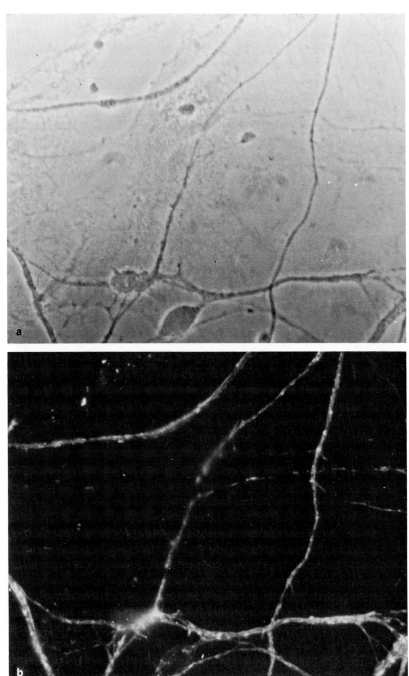

would be unlikely unless a number of surface molecules were restricted in expression to neurons derived on the one hand from the neural tube, or on the other hand from the neural crest or neural placodes.

The methods used for making and testing monoclonal antibodies against neuronal cell surface antigens are described in more detail in the following two subsections.

3.4.1.   A Cell Surface Antigen Present on the Surface of CNS Neurons but Absent from Peripheral Neurons Defined by a Monoclonal Antibody, A4. A monoclonal antibody that reacts with an antigen present on the surface of all rat neurons so far examined which have their cell bodies within the CNS has been defined by Cohen and Selvendran (1981). They immunized a BALB/c mouse twice with cells from 5- to 6-day rat cerebellum in culture highly enriched for granule cell neurons, and took spleen cells from the mouse and fused them with myeloma P3/NS1/1-Ag4-1 using polyethylene glycol (Galfre *et al.*, 1977). Hybridomas were screened for antibody production against cerebellar neurons both by radioimmunoassay of cultured living cerebellar cells and by indirect immunofluorescence. A hybridoma producing antibodies that bound to the surface of cerebellar neurons was selected and cloned twice by limiting dilution (Bartlett *et al.*, 1981) (Fig. 6).

Using tetanus toxin as a neuronal marker to check the distribution of antibody in double-labeling experiments it was found that this antibody binds to an antigen present on the surface of all tetanus toxin$^+$ neurons in dissociated cell cultures of 5- to 6-day rat cerebellum, and neonatal spinal cord, retina, hippocampus, cerebrum, and olfactory bulb. In contrast, tetanus toxin$^+$ neurons in cultures of neonatal rat DRG, SCGs and nodose ganglia do not label with the antibody. However, this antigen is also present at lower levels on some astrocytes, including tetanus toxin$^+$ astrocytes in optic nerve (Raff *et al.*, 1979), and on ciliated ependymal cells. The antigen is absent from all other cells in both CNS and PNS cultures.

Quantitative absorption assays show that the antigen first appears in the rat embryo at day 10 and reaches maximal adult levels soon after birth. It is also present in human, sheep, and rabbit brain but is absent from guinea pig, mouse, chick, and frog brain.

The antigen can be visualized *in situ*. In frozen tissue sections of

---

Figure 6. Cerebellar neurons labeled with A4 monoclonal antibody. Cells in a culture of 5-day old rat cerebellum were labeled with A4 antibody followed by goat anti-MIgRd. Cells were viewed with phase contrast (a) and rhodamine (b) optics. Note that only the neurons, including the cell body at the bottom of the field but none of the flat background cells, are labeled.

16-day rat cerebellum, a germinal layer containing many proliferating neuroblasts still persists (Altman, 1972) and most of the cells in this layer bind the antibody by indirect immunofluorescence. In frozen tissue sections from adult cerebellum the antigen is associated with both the cell bodies and processes of Purkinje cells, basket cells, and granule cells, while white matter shows some weakly positive areas. Frozen tissue sections from adult rat DRG treated with the antibody are completely negative by immunofluorescence.

Cells in cultures from the ENU-derived rat nervous system tumor cell line B104 (Schubert et al., 1974), the rat pheochromocytoma cell line PC12 (Greene and Tischler, 1976) and the rat–mouse glioma–neuroblastoma hybrid NG108 (Nelson et al., 1976) do not bind the A4 antibody.

All the evidence suggests, therefore, that A4 monoclonal antibody recognizes an antigen present on all CNS neurons but absent from PNS neurons.

3.4.2. *A Cell Surface Antigen Present on the Surface of PNS Neurons but Absent from the Surface of CNS Neurons Defined by a Monoclonal Antibody, 38/D7.* A monoclonal antibody that recognizes an antigen with a reciprocal distribution to that described for A4 has also been made (Vulliamy et al., 1981). The antigen is present on the surface of all rat neurons which have their cell bodies originating in the PNS.

Cells from 2-week cultures of 5- to 6-day rat DRG, enriched for neurons, were used to immunize a BALB/c mouse twice. Spleen cells from this mouse were fused with the myeloma P3/NS1/1-Ag4-1 using polyethylene glycol (Galfre et al., 1977), and hybridomas were screened for antibody production against DRG surface antigens by indirect immunofluorescence on living rat DRG cultures grown for 2–14 days in vitro. A hybrid-secreting antibody 38/D7 that bound to the surface of DRG neurons was selected and cloned twice by limiting dilution on layers of peritoneal macrophages (Bartlett et al., 1981) (Fig. 7).

Using tetanus toxin as a neuronal marker to check the distribution of monoclonal antibody, it was found that 38/D7 antibody recognizes an antigen present on all tetanus toxin$^+$ neurons in cultures of 5- to 6-day rat DRG, SCG, nodose ganglion, and myenteric plexus. In addition, in cultures of adrenal medulla, the antigen was present on the surface of norepinephrine-containing cells with the morphology of chromaffin cells. It is also present on the surface of cells of the PC12 pheochromocytoma line, derived originally from a rat adrenal medullary tumor (Greene and Tischler, 1976).

The antigen first appears in ontogeny in 15-day embryonic DRG

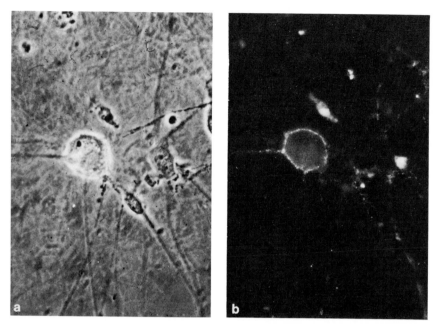

Figure 7. DRG neuron labeled with 38/D7 monoclonal antibody. Cells in a culture of 5-
to 6-day rat DRG were labeled with 38/D7 antibody, followed by goat anti-MIgRd. Cells
were viewed with phase contrast (a) and rhodamine (b) optics. Note clear labeling of the
neuronal cell body and the unstained background cells.

cultures examined by indirect immunofluorescence 24 hr after plating,
or in 14-day DRG embryo cultures examined after 48 hr. It is absent
from neurons of 13-day DRG embryo cultures examined after 48 hr, and
from neurons of 14-day DRG embryo cultures examined after 24 hr.
When first detected in ontogeny the binding of the antibody is very
weak and only present on some neurons; maximal expression on all
neurons appears to develop around the time of birth.

Among CNS cultures tested, at a variety of times varying from 3
days to 30 days after plating, tetanus toxin$^+$ neurons in cultures from
5- to 6-day rat cerebellum, 10-day rat embryo cerebrum, 15-day rat embryo spinal cord, and newborn rat retina were all unlabeled by 38/D7
antibody. The rat ENU-derived tumor cell lines B35, B50, B82, and B104,
all of CNS origin (Schubert et al., 1974), do not bind antibody, and
neither does the rat–mouse glioma–neuroblastoma hybrid NG108 (Nelson et al., 1976).

None of the nonneuronal cells in any of the CNS or PNS cultures bind the antibody, except for a very small number of flat cells in some older cultures; myoblasts and myotubes in primary muscle cultures and melanocytes in skin cultures are also negative.

The distribution of the antigen has been confirmed *in situ* using paraformaldehyde-fixed frozen sections and the indirect immunoperoxidase technique. Visualization in sections of the binding of antibodies to antigens present at fairly low levels on the cell surface is often difficult, but it is possible to see weak labeling of the edge of DRG neuronal cell bodies with 38/D7 antibody. No labeling of neurons or other cells is seen in cerebellar sections.

The low levels of binding obtained using both immunofluorescence and immunoperoxidase techniques have precluded the use of quantitative assays and absorption assays to characterize the tissue distribution of the antigen.

The antigen is probably present only in rat, since in DRG cultures from human, mouse, and chick there is no neuronal labeling. The evidence suggests that the antibody recognizes a neuronal antigen present on all PNS neurons but absent from CNS neurons.

4. APPLICATIONS

Once reliable immunological methods for distinguishing cells in a variety of nervous system cultures had been established they could be used to study problems in several areas of cellular neurobiology. Some of these are described below.

4.1. *Schwann Cell Purification*

Since one of the goals had always been to use immunological methods to separate different cell types, the preparation of populations of pure Schwann cells achieved by Brockes *et al.* (1979) represented an important step forward. Schwann cells were obtained from dissociated newborn rat sciatic nerve. As described earlier in this chapter, the only cell types present in these cultures were Schwann cells, expressing Ran-1 antigen and fibroblasts expressing the Thy-1 antigen (Brockes *et al.*, 1977). Fibroblasts, which initially represent about 50% of the cells, divide at a much faster rate than the Schwann cells. Therefore, treating the cultures with the mitotic poison cytosine arabinoside preferentially kills fibroblasts, leaving cultures which consist of 80–90% pure Schwann cells. Following this, cells are incubated in suspension with anti-Thy-1 serum and complement to eliminate the remaining fibroblasts. When

monitored after this treatment by double-fluorochrome immunofluorescence with antibodies to Thy-1 and Ran-1, over 99.5% of the cells
in cultures are Schwann cells.

The rate of cell division in the purified Schwann cell cultures is low,
but mitosis can be induced by addition of either cholera toxin or an
extract of bovine pituitary and brain (Brockes *et al.*, 1979). The active
factor in these extracts, partially characterized by Raff *et al.* (1978*b*) as
being distinct from fibroblast growth factor and any of the known pituitary hormones, has recently been purified by Brockes *et al.* (1980*a*)
and named glial growth factor.

Thus, by using a combination of mitotic poisons, complement-dependent antibody cytotoxicity and a growth factor to induce cell division,
it proved possible to obtain reasonably large numbers of Schwann cells
for biochemical and other studies (Brockes and Raff, 1979; Brockes *et al.*,
1980*a,b*). An alternative method of obtaining homogeneous populations
of Schwann cells (starting with DRG explants) that does not involve the
use of antibodies has been devised by Wood (1976).

Two conditions are obviously important in using antibodies as negative selection agents for cell purification, and these are not always easy
to realize in practice. First, the cytotoxic antibodies used must alone, or
in combination, recognize all the cell types in the culture except the one
of interest; second, it is important to have a mitogenic factor which will
induce the remaining cells to divide at a reasonable rate after purification. Cells such as oligodendrocytes, which represent <5% cells in cultures of optic nerve or corpus callosum (Raff *et al.*, 1979), are probably
better purified by alternative methods (McCarthy and de Vellis, 1980).

So far the use of antibodies for positive selection, using methods
such as the FACS, have not been widely exploited for separation of
nervous system cells, but they are almost certainly more suitable for
purification of cells representing small numbers in the original population and will undoubtedly be used more in the future.

4.2. Comparison between the Properties of Myelin-Specific Glycolipids and Proteins in Rat Oligodendrocytes and Schwann Cells in Culture

The two major myelin glycolipids, GalC and sulfatide, are normally
expressed by oligodendrocytes in nonmyelinating CNS cultures for a
period of many weeks. Paradoxically, they are not normally expressed
by Schwann cells in nonmyelinating sciatic nerve or DRG cultures (Raff
et al., 1978*a*).

Schwann cells *in situ* begin to make immunochemically detectable
amounts of the peripheral myelin basic proteins (P_1 and P_2) and the

major glycoprotein P_0 at the time of onset of myelination, which is between birth and 5 days in the rat (Brockes *et al.*, 1980*a*), so that initially it was surprising to find that GalC is not expressed by Schwann cells in sciatic nerve cultures from newborn to 5-day animals. Further experiments (Mirsky *et al.*, 1980) showed that approximately 50% of cells from trypsin-dissociated newborn sciatic nerve are $GalC^+$, while 20–30% of a nonoverlapping population of cells are $Thy-1^+$ fibroblasts. When sciatic nerve or DRG cultures are examined by double-fluorochrome indirect immunofluorescence 16 hr after plating, 25–55% of the Schwann cells express detectable amounts of both Ran-1 and GalC on their surface (Fig. 8). A similar proportion of the Schwann cells also express sulfatide. However, the proportion of $Ran-1^+$ Schwann cells in sciatic nerve or DRG cultures labeled by anti-GalC or antisulfatide antibodies decreases progressively with time in culture, so that by 72 hr only rare cells express these glycolipids. In comparable cultures from the SCG and the sympathetic postganglionic nerve trunk, where the number of myelinated axons is normally very low, only 1% of the $Ran-1^+$ Schwann cells express GalC on their surface after 16 hr in culture.

When oligodendrocytes and Schwann cells are compared with respect to expression of some of the major myelin proteins a similar picture emerges. Oligodendrocytes from 5-day rat optic nerve cultures which are making GalC, also make myelin basic protein for many weeks in culture even when no neurons are present (Fig. 9). Basic protein is not detectable on the surface but after fixation can be seen most intensely in the cell bodies and also extending into some of the processes. By contrast, in Schwann cells the myelin basic protein P_1 and peripheral myelin glycoprotein P_0 are initially expressed in a small proportion of fixed cells in 16 hr cultures of newborn to 5-day sciatic nerve or DRG, but gradually disappear when cells are examined over the next 3 days in culture. The staining is usually confined to one or two vesicles near the nucleus (Fig. 10). Schwann cells derived from the SCG and trunk do not express P_1 or P_0.

When oligodendrocytes and Schwann cells are compared with respect to the first developmental appearance of GalC, sulfatide, and myelin proteins, more information can be obtained. In rat optic nerve, myelination begins at around 6 days after birth (Skoff *et al.*, 1976). In cultures of newborn optic nerve examined by immunofluorescence after 24 hr, $GalC^+$ oligodendrocytes do not make detectable amounts of basic protein. However, when such cultures are reexamined 6 days after plating, the $GalC^+$ oligodendrocytes are now making basic protein, even though the cultures are devoid of neurons.

A few Schwann cells expressing GalC on their surface can first be

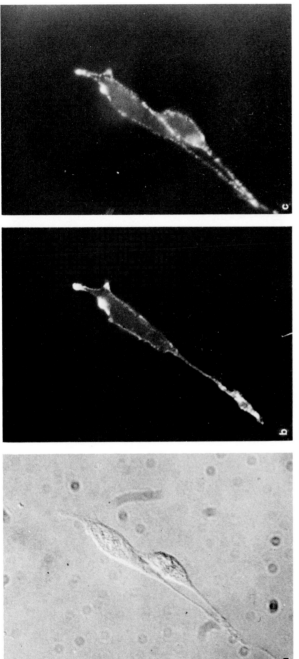

Figure 8. GalC$^+$ and GalC$^-$ Schwann cells. Two Schwann cells in a culture of newborn sciatic nerve were labeled after 16–20 hr with mouse anti-Ran-1 and rabbit anti-GalC followed by a mixture of goat anti-MIgRd and goat anti-RIgFl. Cells were viewed with Nomarski (a), rhodamine (b), and fluorescein (c) optics.

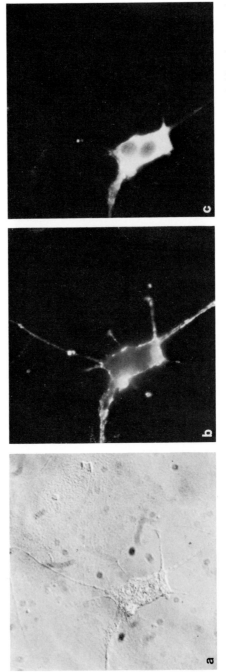

Figure 9. GalC$^+$, basic protein$^+$ oligodendrocyte. Cells in cultures of 5- to 6-day rat optic nerve, labeled with rabbit anti-GalC and goat-anti-RIgRd, fixed and incubated with guinea pig anti-basic protein and goat anti-guinea pig Ig fluorescein. Cells were viewed with Nomarski (a), rhodamine (b), and fluorescein (c) optics.

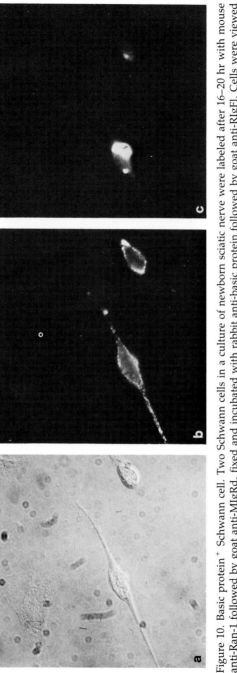

Figure 10. Basic protein⁺ Schwann cell. Two Schwann cells in a culture of newborn sciatic nerve were labeled after 16–20 hr with mouse anti-Ran-1 followed by goat anti-MIgRd, fixed and incubated with rabbit anti-basic protein followed by goat anti-RIgFl. Cells were viewed with Nomarski (a), rhodamine (b), and fluorescein (c) optics. Two Schwann cells, but not the fibroblastic cell, are Ran-1⁺, and one of these is basic protein⁺.

detected in 16 hr-sciatic nerve or DRG cultures from 19-day-embryo rats. At this stage no P_1 or P_0 positive cells are found and no detectable amounts are made over a week in culture. In the sciatic nerve of newborn animals taken within 14 hr of birth, at a time when less than 1% of all Schwann cells in comparable sciatic nerves examined in the electron microscope are myelinating, 20–35% of the Schwann cells express GalC and sulfatide and none of these contain P_0 and P_1 or P_2. In cultures made from 1-day sciatic nerves, when myelination has begun in a significant proportion of axons, 5–8% of the Schwann cells contain P_0 or P_1 and 2% were positive for P_2. In 5- to 7-day rat sciatic nerve or DRG, at a time when myelination is proceeding rapidly (Webster, 1971), 40–60% of Schwann cells are $GalC^+$; of these, 34–50% are $P_0{}^+$, 9–38% are $P_1{}^+$, and 7–11% are $P_2{}^+$ (Mirsky et al., 1980; Winter et al., 1982). Thus it seems that the myelin glycolipids are synthesized in immuno-histochemically detectable amounts well before the wrapping associated with myelination begins, whereas the myelin proteins are not detectable until myelination begins, suggesting that the synthesis of glycolipids is an important step which precedes myelination.

Thus oligodendrocytes synthesize both myelin glycolipids and proteins in culture without requiring the continued presence of neurons, with synthesis beginning well before the onset of myelination. Schwann cells behave differently, perhaps reflecting the fact that in the peripheral nervous system they serve at least two functions. They ensheath but do not myelinate smaller axons and ensheath and myelinate larger axons. Schwann cells taken from nerves where few axons are myelinated do not normally express immunohistochemically detectable amounts of the major myelin glycolipids or proteins, whereas Schwann cells taken from nerves where myelination is occurring initially possess GalC, sulfatide, P_0, and P_1, but lose them with time in culture. These results suggest that, in contrast to oligodendrocytes, Schwann cells require contact with axons which are capable of inducing myelination for induction and continuing synthesis of high levels of the myelin glycolipids and proteins.

Sternberger et al. (1978a,b) have reported previously that in neonatal rat brain sections, basic protein, visualized using immunoperoxidase techniques, can be detected in the oligodendrocyte cytoplasm before morphological myelin sheath formation has begun. In sections, GalC, by contrast, can only be detected associated with the myelin sheath and is not seen on the surface of the oligodendrocyte cell body. In culture (Mirsky et al., 1980) GalC and sulfatide are detectable on the surface of oligodendrocytes earlier in ontogeny than basic protein and in Schwann cells earlier than either the peripheral glycoprotein P_0 or the basic protein

P_1, suggesting that glycolipid synthesis may precede the synthesis of myelin proteins.

The fact that rat Schwann cells stop making detectable amounts of myelin-specific glycolipids and proteins in culture means that these molecules can serve as convenient immunological markers for studying events connected with Schwann cell myelination *in vitro*.

4.3. The Use of Cell-Type-Specific Markers to Investigate the Development of Neurons, Astrocytes, Ependymal Cells, and Oligodendrocytes in Dissociated Cell Cultures from Embryonic Rat Brain

When antibodies to tetanus toxin, GFAP, Ran-2, and GalC are used to study the development of the major classes of cells in dissociated cell cultures from 10-day embryonic rat brain, and their appearance over time in cultures is compared with their appearance in embryological development, it is found that the major classes of glial cells develop at the same time *in vitro* and *in vivo* (Abney *et al.*, 1981). This important conclusion suggests that astrocytes, ependymal cells, and oligodendrocytes can develop from their precursor cells in mixed dissociated cultures without requiring constant positional information (Wolpert, 1969) from neighboring cells. Furthermore, it implies either that they acquire this type of information prior to the 10th embryonic day or that they do not require it for differentiation. Since these studies involve mixed cultures, it is still possible that the cooperative presence of several cell types is required for proper differentiation of individual glial cells, and it should be possible to use antibodies to determine whether this is so.

Tetanus toxin$^+$ small neurons are detected in large numbers by immunofluorescence after 24–72 hr in such cultures (see Table II). With time, the size and shape of the neuronal cell bodies became more variable and the processes form a dense network over the surface of the culture. When cultures are exposed to [^{3}H]thymidine after 3 or 7 days *in vitro* to detect dividing cells, no tetanus toxin$^+$ cells have incorporated [^{3}H] thymidine. After 2 weeks in culture a small proportion of tetanus toxin$^+$ neurons develop Thy-1 on their surface, an observation consistent with previous results (Mirsky and Thompson, 1975; Currie *et al.*, 1977).

Although flat, fibroblastic-looking cells are present from the earliest times in 10-day embryonic brain cultures, none contain detectable amounts of the astrocyte marker GFAP until after 5–6 days in culture. At 5–6 days, small numbers of GFAP$^+$ cells are seen with GFAP$^+$ filament bundles extending into one or two long processes. From this time onward the number of GFAP$^+$ cells increases steadily and by 2

Table II. Times of Appearance of Neural Cells in Vivo and in Dissociated Cell Cultures of 10- or 13-Day Embryonic Rat Brain[a]

| | | | Time of first appearance | |
| | | | In vitro (days) | |
Cell type	Marker	In vivo[b] (days)	10-day embryo	13-day embryo
Neurons	Tetanus toxin receptors	11	1	1
Macrophages	Fc receptors	11	1	1
Astrocyte precursors	Ran-2$^+$, GFAP$^-$	11	1	1
Astrocytes	GFAP	15–16	5–6	2–3
Ependymal cells	Beating cilia	17–18	7–8	4–5
Oligodendrocytes	GalC	2–3 after birth[c]	13–14	10–11

[a] From Abney et al. (1981).
[b] Cells were studied in freshly prepared suspensions of brain.
[c] Day of birth (gestation period = 21 days) is considered day 0.

weeks large areas of the culture are covered with an interwoven network of GFAP$^+$ processes. Most of the GFAP$^+$ cells are also Ran-2$^+$, but none are labeled with tetanus toxin or antibodies against GalC, Thy-1, or fibronectin even after 6 weeks in culture. This result is somewhat surprising, since as mentioned earlier (Section 1.3), some GFAP$^+$ astrocytes in cultures from neonatal cerebellum and corpus callosum develop Thy-1 after 1 week in culture (Pruss, 1979). A proportion of the GFAP$^+$ astrocytes in these embryonic cultures are dividing. In suspensions prepared from embryo cerebrum, GFAP$^+$ cells are first detected in 15- to 16-day embryos. This is 2 days earlier than in a previous study using embryonic mouse brain (Kozak et al., 1978).

After only 24 hr in culture some of the flat cells are weakly Ran-2$^+$. The number of Ran-2$^+$ cells and the surface concentration of the antigen, visualized by indirect immunofluorescence, increase progressively with time in culture. At 6–7 days in culture, Ran 2$^+$, GFAP$^+$ astrocytes are first seen, and over the next few days the proportion of Ran 2$^+$, GFAP$^-$ cells declines while the proportion of Ran 2$^+$, GFAP$^+$ cells increases, until by 2 weeks in culture most Ran 2$^+$ cells are also GFAP$^+$, suggesting that some Ran 2$^+$, GFAP$^-$ cells might be astrocyte precursors.

To determine whether this is so, the following experiment was done. Four-day cultures of 10d embryonic rat brain, devoid of GFAP$^+$ astrocytes, are incubated for 2 hr with monoclonal antibodies against Ran-2 and maintained in culture for a further 2 or 3 days. They are then incubated with goat anti-MIgRd visualize any residual Ran-2 antibodies, fixed and incubated with rabbit anti-GFAP, and goat anti-RIgF1. More than 90% of the differentiated astrocytes which expressed GFAP also have residual Ran-2 antibodies on their surface. It is therefore concluded that the majority of astrocyte precursors are Ran-2$^+$.

Oligodendrocytes develop relatively late *in vivo*, and GalC-positive cells are first detected in freshly prepared suspensions from the cerebrum in 2- to 3-day rats. Similarly, in cultures from 10-day embryo brain, GalC$^+$ oligodendrocytes do not develop until the equivalent time of the 13th–14th day in culture. They are normally found on top of a dense monolayer of flat cells, have dark nuclei and cytoplasm, and often have branched processes. Fewer than 5% of GalC$^+$ oligodendrocytes in 14- to 15-day cultures were dividing when measured by [^{3}H]thymidine uptake.

Macrophages, which bind normal IgG through Fc receptors and phagocytose latex beads, are present in 10-day embryonic brain cultures as early as 24 hr after plating. Whether they are endogenous macrophages (microglial cells) or are derived from contaminating blood is uncertain.

Ependymal cells, detected by their beating cilia and the presence of the Ran-2 surface antigen, are first seen after 7–8 days in culture, and in increasing numbers on subsequent days. In freshly prepared suspensions from embryo cerebrum they are first detected at the equivalent time of 17–18 days.

When dissociated cell cultures are made from 13-day embryonic brain, all the glial-cell-type-specific markers develop 3 days earlier than in the 10-day embryonic cultures.

Thus, it has proved possible to use cell-type-specific markers to study the development of the major nervous system cell types in CNS embryonic cultures, to follow the appearance of one cell type, the astrocyte, from a precursor cell by the use of two markers in combination, and to show that after embryonic day 10 the appearance of the cells parallels that observed *in vivo*.

4.4. Cell Surface Markers Can Be Used to Identify Human Glial and Neuronal Cells in Culture

Ethical considerations preclude the use of living human tissue *in situ* to any great extent for the investigation of disease. Therefore, there is a clear need to develop reliable methods for the study of normal human cells in tissue culture. In the nervous system, in particular, the effects of viruses, toxins, antibodies, or even cytotoxic lymphocytes on particular cell types might be investigated in this way.

A good example of this approach has been the use of human and rat muscle cultures to study the effects of antibodies from patients with myasthenia gravis or animals with experimental autoimmune myasthenia gravis on acetylcholine receptor turnover (Heinemann et al., 1977; Bevan et al., 1977).

In many experiments it is clearly important to be able to distinguish the different cell types being cultured since viruses, toxins, and antibodies may well attack one cell type and not another. Kennedy et al. (1980) used dissociated cell cultures from 15- to 21-week human fetal optic nerve, spinal cord, DRG, and leptomeninges to investigate whether the cell-type-specific markers previously used in rat nervous system cultures could also be used in human cultures.

Originally, GFAP was isolated from human brain (Eng et al., 1971), and anti-human GFAP serum was used to show that it was present in astrocytes from human adult and fetal brain in frozen tissue sections (Bignami et al., 1972; Bignami and Dahl, 1974) and also in explant cultures (Antanitus et al., 1975). It was therefore unsurprising to find that GFAP is also present in astrocytes in dissociated cell cultures of human fetal optic nerve and spinal cord. Contrary to a previous report that cultured human astrocytes make fibronectin [but where the astrocytes were not positively identified by the presence of GFAP (Vaheri et al., 1976)], no GFAP$^+$ astrocytes expressing fibronectin are found. However, in a manner analogous to astrocytes in neonatal rat cerebellum and corpus callosum (Pruss, 1979) some of the GFAP$^+$ astrocytes also express the human Thy-1 antigen on their surface.

In human fetal DRG cultures tetanus toxin binds only to neurons, which are distinguished by their large refractile cell bodies and long processes. No viable neurons are in the spinal cord cultures, but the toxin does not bind to any other cell type in either spinal cord, optic nerve, or leptomeningeal cultures. In double-fluorochrome immunofluorescence experiments all of the tetanus toxin$^+$ neurons in the DRG also express the human Thy-1 antigen on their surface. This is comparable to rat DRG, where all tetanus toxin$^+$ neurons also express the Thy-1 antigen (Fields et al., 1978).

About 4% of cells in optic nerve and spinal cord cultures show surface labelling with anti-GalC serum for up to 1 week in culture. These cells are presumably oligodendrocytes since their morphology is similar to that seen in rat CNS cultures. They are not labeled with anti-GFAP, tetanus toxin, anti-human Thy-1, or antifibronectin sera. In the spinal cord cultures about 50% of the GalC$^+$ oligodendrocytes also stain with antibasic protein serum, but in the optic nerve cultures none of the GalC$^+$ oligodendrocytes make basic protein. This may reflect the later onset of myelination in optic nerve compared with spinal cord.

Some of the Schwann cells in human fetal DRG cultures can be identified by their typical bipolar morphology. None of these cells express either the Ran-1 antigen or the human Thy-1 antigen. Therefore Ran-1 cannot be used as a marker for human Schwann cells. However, when the cultures are examined 16 hr after plating for the presence of GalC, about 25% of the bipolar cells show intense surface labeling with anti-GalC serum, and about 30% of these cells also contain the myelin basic protein P_1 and the glycoprotein P_0 in the typical vesicular form seen in rat Schwann cells. Expression of GalC, P_1, and P_0 decline with time in culture, as in the rat, and by 96 hr very few cells are positive for any of these antigens.

A large proportion of the flat cells in human fetal DRG, spinal cord, optic nerve, and leptomeningeal cultures are GFAP$^-$. In all cultures more than 95% of these cells are fibronectin$^+$. In DRG and spinal cord cultures more than 80% of these cells express the human Thy-1 antigen and are thus likely to be fibroblasts, while in leptomeningeal and optic nerve cultures few cells do. Therefore, it seems likely that most of these cells are leptomeningeal.

Macrophages, which ingest latex particles and bind IgG through their Fc receptors, are found in all cultures, though less frequently in those from DRG.

Thus, with the exception of Ran-1, and the substitution of anti-human Thy-1 serum for mouse anti-Thy-1.1 serum, all of the specific markers used to identify the major cell types in rat nervous system cultures can also be used in human nervous system cultures. In addition, the differences in expression of the myelin glycolipid and proteins between oligodendrocytes and Schwann cells previously observed and commented on in the neonatal rat (Mirsky et al., 1980) also hold true in the case of human oligodendrocytes and Schwann cells.

5. CONCLUSIONS

Using antibodies and tetanus toxin it has been possible to devise a series of cell-type-specific markers to distinguish the major cell types in nervous system cultures. Obviously, other antigens specific to the major cell types could have been chosen, but the markers described here have proved themselves, on the whole, easy and reliable to use. With the exception of Schwann cells, which can only be defined antigenically in rat, the antibodies and toxin can be used to define the major nervous system cell types in rat, mouse, human, and chick.

Furthermore, as outlined in this chapter, these markers have already proved valuable as tools in a number of different areas of cellular neurobiology. For instance, the characterization of monoclonal antibodies to different cell subpopulations is made immeasurably easier by use of the major cell type markers in conjunction with double-fluorochrome immunofluorescence, and the purification of Schwann cells is more effective when Thy-1 antibody and complement is used in conjunction with cytosine arabinoside to eliminate fibroblasts. In comparing the properties of oligodendrocytes and Schwann cells with respect to expression of myelin glycolipids and proteins, the markers are essential and they have proved invaluable for studying the development of glial cells in culture.

A comparison with the wide and often unexpected horizons which have opened up in immunology by the use of techniques similar to those described here suggest caution in predicting the most promising areas for future research. However, a few obvious possibilities come to mind. Development of a wider range of monoclonal antibodies to subpopulations of neurons and glia should allow correlations of surface with intracellular properties and help elucidate the differences between the surface characteristics of CNS and PNS neurons. They should also provide information at a molecular level about functionally important molecules in the nervous system, particularly those involved in recognition and interaction between different cells. In particular, it should be possible to use antibodies to perturb development *in vitro* and *in vivo* in a variety of ways. Another area where these techniques could be important is in studies of cellular ontogeny in the developing nervous system, where there is a need for antibodies to antigens which enable cell lineages to be traced more effectively than the present morphological and autoradiographic methods allow. A promising start in this direction has been made by Schmechel and Rakic (1979*a*,*b*), who have used a combination of morphological and autoradiographic techniques in combination with antibodies to GFAP to follow the development of radial glial cells in monkey cerebrum through their transformation into astrocytes and ependymal cells. In the rat, it should be possible to use the presence of the Ran-2 antigen on both GFAP$^-$ astrocyte precursors and GFAP$^+$ astrocytes and to use the monoclonal antibody A4, which recognizes an antigen present on both neuroblasts and neurons, to study the rules which govern the transition of the precursor into the more mature cell type. (An account of new markers for precursors to oligodendrocytes is given in Chapter 7.) However, at present no markers distinguish between nonmyelinating Schwann and satellite cells and their precursors.

The goal of understanding the detailed interactions of cells in the nervous system is still elusive, but immunological methods have helped to solve some elementary problems and will certainly become more important in the future.

ACKNOWLEDGMENTS

This chapter describes research done in the MRC Neuroimmunology Project, Zoology Department, University College London, over a number of years. I therefore thank all members of the project, past and present, for their work, advice, and encouragement, and especially Martin Raff, Jeremy Brockes, Kay Fields, and Rebecca Pruss.

6. REFERENCES

Akeson, R., and Seeger, R. C., 1977, Interspecies neural membrane antigen on cultured human and murine neuroblastoma cells, *J. Immunol.* **118**:1995.

Abney, E. R., Bartlett, P. P., and Raff, M. C., 1981, Astrocytes, ependymal cells and oligodendrocytes develop on schedule in dissociated cell cultures of embryonic rat brain, *Dev. Biol.* **83**:301.

Altman, J., 1972, Postnatal development of the cerebellar cortex in the rat. I. The external germinal layer, *J. Comp. Neurol.* **145**:465.

Antanitus, D. S., Choi, B. H., Lapham, L. W., 1975, Immunofluorescence staining of astrocytes *in vitro* using antiserum to glial fibrillary acidic protein, *Brain Res.* **89**:363.

Barnstable, C. J., 1980, Monoclonal antibodies which recognize different cell types in the rat retina, *Nature (London)* **286**:231.

Bartlett, P. F., Noble, M. D., Pruss, R. M., Raff, M. C., Rattray, S., and Williams, C. A., 1981, Rat neural antigen-2 (Ran-2): A cell surface antigen on astrocytes, ependymal cells, Müller cells and leptomeninges defined by a monoclonal antibody, *Brain Res.* **204**:339.

Bevan, S., Kullberg, R. W., and Heinemann, S. F., 1977, Human myasthenic sera reduce acetylcholine sensitivity of human muscle cells in tissue culture, *Nature (London)* **267**:263.

Bignami, A., and Dahl, D., 1973, Differentiation of astrocytes in the cerebellar cortex and the pyramidal tracts in the newborn rat. An immunofluorescence study with antibodies to a protein specific to astrocytes, *Brain Res.* **49**:393.

Bignami, A., and Dahl, D., 1974, Astrocyte-specific protein and neuroglial differentiation. An immunofluorescence study with antibodies to glial fibrillary acidic protein, *J. Comp. Neurol.* **153**:27.

Bignami, A., Eng, L. F., Dahl, D., and Uyeda, C. T., 1972, Localization of the glial fibrillary acidic protein in astrocytes by immunofluorescence, *Brain Res.* **43**:429.

Bock, E., Moller, M., Nissen, C., and Sensenbrenner, M., 1977, Glial fibrillary acidic protein in primary astroglial cultures derived from newborn rat brain, *FEBS Lett.* **83**:207.

Brockes, J. P., and Raff, M. C., 1979, Studies on cultured rat Schwann cells. II. Comparison with a rat Schwann cell line, *In vitro*, **15**:772.

Brockes, J. P., Fields, K. L., and Raff, M. C., 1977, A surface antigenic marker for rat Schwann cells, *Nature (London)* **266**:364.

Brockes, J. P., Fields, K. L., and Raff, M. C., 1979, Studies on cultured rat Schwann cells. I. Establishment of purified populations from cultures of peripheral nerve, *Brain Res.* **165**:105.

Brockes, J. P., Raff, M. C., Nishiguchi, D. J., and Winter, J., 1980a, Studies on cultured rat Schwann cells. III. Assays for peripheral myelin proteins, *J. Neurocytol.* **9**:67.

Brockes, J. P., Lemke, G. E., and Balzer, D. R., Jr., 1980b, Purification and preliminary characterization of a glial growth factor from the bovine pituitary, *J. Biol. Chem.* **255**:8374.

Burridge, K., 1978, Direct identification of specific glycoproteins and antigens in sodium dodecyl sulfate gels, in: *Methods in Enzymology*, vol. 50 (S. P. Colowick and N. O. Kaplan, eds.), pp. 54–64, Academic Press, New York.

Cantor, H., and Boyse, E., 1977, Regulation of the immune response by T-cell subclasses, *Contemp. Top. Immunobiol.* **7**:47.

Cohen, J., and Selvendran, S. Y., 1981, A neurone-specific cell-surface antigen in the central nervous system not shared by peripheral neurones, *Nature (London)* **291**:421.

Cook, R. D., and Burnstock, G., 1976, The ultrastructure of Auerbach's plexus in the guinea-pig. II. Non-neuronal elements, *J. Neurocytol.* **5**:195.

Cuello, A. C., Galfre, G., and Milstein, C., 1979, Detection of substance P in the central nervous system by a monoclonal antibody, *Proc. Natl. Acad. Sci. U.S.A.* **76**:3532.

Currie, D. N., Fields, K. L., and Dutton, G. R., 1977, GABA autoradiography and Thy 1.1 immunofluorescent properties of primary cell cultures of postnatal rat cerebellum, *Proc. Int. Soc. Neurochem.* **6**:635.

Dahl, D., and Bignami, A., 1976, Immunogenic properties of the glial fibrillary acidic protein, *Brain Res.* **116**:150.

Dimpfel, W., Neale, J. H., and Habermann, E., 1975, ^{125}I-labelled tetanus toxin as a neuronal marker in tissue cultures derived from embryonic CNS, *Naunyn-Schmiedebergs Arch. Exp. Pathol. Pharmakol.* **290**:329.

Eisenbarth, G. S., Walsh, F. S., and Nirenberg, M., 1979, Monoclonal antibody to a plasma membrane antigen of neurons, *Proc. Natl. Acad. Sci. U.S.A.* **76**:4913.

Eng, L. F., Vanderhaegen, J. J., Bignami, A., and Gerstl, B., 1971, An acidic protein isolated from fibrous astrocytes, *Brain Res.* **28**:351.

Fields, K. L., Gosling, C., Megson, M., and Stern, P. L., 1975, New cell surface antigens in rat defined by tumors of the nervous system, *Proc. Natl. Acad. Sci. U.S.A.* **72**:1286.

Fields, K. L., Brockes, J. P., Mirsky, R., and Wendon, L. M. B., 1978, Cell surface markers for distinguishing different types of rat dorsal root ganglion cells in culture, *Cell* **14**:43.

Fleischhauer, K., 1972, Ependymal and sub-ependymal layer, in: *The Structure and Function of Nervous Tissue*, vol. 6 (G. H. Bourne, ed.), pp. 1–46, Academic Press, New York.

Gabella, G., 1972, Fine structure of the myenteric plexus in the guinea-pig ileum, *J. Anat.* **111**:69.

Galfre, G., Howe, S. C., Milstein, C., Butcher, G. W., and Howard, J. C., 1977, Antibodies to major histocompatibility antigens produced by hybrid cell lines, *Nature (London)* **266**:550.

Gilbert, D. S., Newby, B. J., and Anderton, B. H., 1975, Neurofilament disguise, destruction and discipline, *Nature (London)* **256**:586.

Greene, L. A., and Tischler, A. S., 1976, Establishment of a noradrenergic clonal line of rat adrenal pheochromocytoma cells which respond to nerve growth factor, *Proc. Natl. Acad. Sci. U.S.A.* **73**:2424.

Heinemann, S., Bevan, S., Kullberg, R., Lindstrom, J., and Rice, J., 1977, Modulation of acetylcholine receptor by antibody against the receptor, *Proc. Natl. Acad. Sci. U.S.A.* **74:**3090.

Hoffman, P. N., and Lasek, R. J., 1975, The slow component of axonal transport. Identification of major structural polypeptides of the axon and their generality among mammalian neurons, *J. Cell Biol.* **66:**351.

Hynes, R. O., 1973, Alteration of cell-surface proteins by viral transformation and proteolysis, *Proc. Natl. Acad. Sci. U.S.A.* **70:**3170.

Jessen, K. R., and Mirsky, R., 1980, Glial cells in the enteric nervous system contain glial fibrillary acidic protein, *Nature (London)* **286:**736.

Kennedy, P. G. E., Lisak, R. P., and Raff, M. C., 1980, Cell type-specific markers for human glial and neuronal cells in culture, *Lab. Invest.* **43:**342.

Kennett, R. H., and Gilbert, F., 1979, Hybrid myelomas producing antibodies against a human neuroblastoma antigen present on fetal brain, *Science* **203:**1120.

Köhler, G., and Milstein, C., 1975, Continuous cultures of fused cells secreting antibody of predefined specificity, *Nature (London)* **256:**495.

Kozak, L. P., Dahl, D., and Bignami, A., 1978, Glial fibrillary acidic protein in reaggregating and monolayer cultures of fetal mouse cerebral hemispheres, *Brain Res.* **150:**631.

Lagenaur, C., Sommer, I., and Schachner, M., 1980, Subclass of astroglia in mouse cerebellum recognized by monoclonal antibody, *Dev. Biol.* **79:**367.

Lazarides, E., 1980, Intermediate filaments as mechanical integrators of cellular space, *Nature (London)* **283:**249.

Ledbetter, J. A., and Herzenberg, L. A., 1979, Xenogeneic monoclonal antibodies to mouse lymphoid differentiation antigens, *Immunological Rev.* **47:**63.

McCarthy, K. D., and de Vellis, J., 1980, Preparation of separate astroglial and oligodendroglial cultures from rat cerebral tissue, *J. Cell Biol.* **85:**890.

Mirsky, R., and Thompson, E. J., 1975, Thy-1 (theta) antigen on the surface of morphologically distinct brain cell types, *Cell* **4:**95.

Mirsky, R, Wendon, L. M. B., Black, P., Stolkin, C., and Bray, D., 1978, Tetanus toxin: A cell surface marker for neurones in culture, *Brain Res.* **148:**251.

Mirsky, R., Winter, J., Abney, E. R., Pruss, R. M., Gavrilovic, J., and Raff, M. C., 1980, Myelin-specific proteins and glycolipids in rat Schwann cells and oligodendrocytes in culture, *J. Cell Biol.* **84:**483.

Nelson, P., Clifford, C., and Nirenberg, M., 1976, Synapse formation between clonal neuroblastoma X glioma hybrid cells and striated muscle cells, *Proc. Natl. Acad. Sci. U.S.A.* **73:**123.

Osborn, M., Franke, W. W., and Weber, K., 1980, Direct demonstration of the presence of two immunologically distinct intermediate-sized filament systems in the same cell by double immunofluorescence microscopy, *Exp. Cell Res.* **125:**37.

Parkhouse, R. M. E., and Cooper, M. D., 1977, A model for the differentiation of B lymphocytes with implications for the biological role of IgD, *Immunol. Rev.* **37:**105.

Pruss, R., 1979, Thy-1 antigen on astrocytes in long-term cultures of rat central nervous system, *Nature (London)* **280:**688.

Pruss, R. M., Mirsky, R., Raff, M. C., Thorpe, R., Dowding, A. J., and Anderton, B. H., 1981, All classes of intermediate filaments share a common antigenic determinant defined by a monoclonal antibody, *Cell* (December issue).

Raff, M. C., 1970, Two distinct populations of peripheral lymphocytes in mice distinguishable by immunofluorescence, *Immunology* **19:**637.

Raff, M. C., Mirsky, R., Fields, K. L., Lisak, R. P., Dorfman, S. H., Silberberg, D. H.,

Gregson, N. A., Leibowitz, S., and Kennedy, M. C., 1978a, Galactocerebroside is a specific cell-surface antigenic marker for oligodendrocytes in culture, *Nature (London)* **274**:813.

Raff, M. C., Abney, E. R., Hornby-Smith, A., and Brockes, J. P., 1978b, Schwann cell growth factors, *Cell* **15**:813.

Raff, M. C., Fields, K. L., Hakomori, S.-I., Mirsky, R., Pruss, R. M., and Winter, J., 1979, Cell-type-specific markers for distinguishing and studying neurons and the major classes of glial cells in culture, *Brain Res.* **174**:283.

Reif, A. E., and Allen, J. M. V., 1964, The AKR thymic antigen and its distribution in leukaemias and nervous tissues, *J. Exp. Med.* **120**:413.

Roslansky, P. F., Cornell-Bell, A., Rice, R. V., and Adelman, W. J., 1980, Polypeptide composition of squid neurofilaments, *Proc. Natl. Acad. Sci. U.S.A.* **77**:404.

Schachner, M., Ruberg, M. Z., and Carnow, T. B., 1976, Histological localization of nervous system antigens in the cerebellum by immunoperoxidase labelling, *Brain Res. Bull.* **1**:367.

Schachner, M., Hedley-Whyte, E. T., Hsu, D. W., Schoonmaker, G., and Bignami, A., 1977, Ultrastructural localization of glial fibrillary acidic protein in mouse cerebellum by immunoperoxidase labelling, *J. Cell Biol.* **75**:67.

Schachner, M., Schoonmaker, G., and Hynes, R. O., 1978, Cellular and subcellular localisation of LETS protein in the nervous system, *Brain Res.* **158**:149.

Schmechel, D. E., and Rakic, P., 1979a, A Golgi study of radial glial cells in developing monkey telencephalon: Morphogenesis and transformation into astrocytes, *Anat. Embryol.* **156**:115.

Schmechel, D. E., and Rakic, P., 1979b, Arrested proliferation of radial glial cells during midgestation in rhesus monkey, *Nature* **277**:303.

Schubert, D., Heinemann, S., Carlisle, W., Tarikas, H., and Kimes, B., 1974, Clonal cell lines from the rat central nervous system, *Nature (London)* **249**:224.

Shantha, T. R., and Bourne, G. H., 1968, The perineural epithelium—a new concept, in: *The Structure and Function of Nervous Tissue*, vol. 1 (G. H. Bourne, ed.), pp. 380–459, Academic Press, New York.

Skoff, R. P., Price, D. L., and Stocks, A., 1976, Electron microscopic autoradiographic studies of gliogenesis in rat optic nerve. II. Time of origin, *J. Comp. Neurol.* **169**:313.

Stallcup, W. B., and Cohn, M., 1976, Correlation of surface antigens and cell type in cloned cell lines from the rat central nervous system, *Exp. Cell Res.* **98**:285.

Steinert, P. M., Idler, W. W., and Goldman, R. D., 1980, Intermediate filaments of baby hamster kidney (BHK-21) cells and bovine epidermal keratinocytes have similar ultrastructures and subunit domain structures, *Proc. Natl. Acad. Sci. U.S.A.* **77**:4534.

Stern, P. L., 1973, Theta alloantigen on mouse and rat fibroblasts, *Nature (London) New Biol.* **246**:76.

Sternberger, N. H., Itoyama, Y., Kies, M. W., and Webster, H. de F., 1978a, Immunochemical method to identify basic protein in myelin-forming oligodendrocytes of newborn rat, *J. Neurocytol.* **7**:251.

Sternberger, N. H., Itoyama, Y., Kies, M. W., and Webster, H. de F., 1978b, Myelin basic protein demonstrated immunochemically in oligodendroglia prior to myelin sheath formation, *Proc. Natl. Acad. Sci. U.S.A.* **75**:2521.

Vaheri, A., Ruoslahti, E., Westermark, B., and Ponten, J., 1976, A common cell-type-specific surface antigen in cultured human glial cells and fibroblasts: Loss in malignant cells, *J. Exp. Med.* **143**:64.

Van Heyningen, W. E., 1963, The fixation of tetanus toxin, strychnine, serotonin and other substances by ganglioside, *J. Gen. Microbiol.* **31**:375.

Vulliamy, T., and Messenger, E. A., 1981, Tetanus toxin: A marker of Amphibian neuronal differentiation *in vitro, Neurosci. Lett.* **22**:87.

Vulliamy, T., Rattray, S., and Mirsky, R., 1981, Sensory and autonomic peripheral neurones express a cell surface antigen not expressed by central neurones, *Nature (London)* **291**:418.

Wang, C., Asai, D. J., and Lazarides, E., 1980, The 68,000-dalton neurofilament-associated polypeptide is a component of non-neuronal cells and of skeletal myofibrils, *Proc. Natl. Acad. Sci. U.S.A.* **77**:1541.

Wartiovaara, J., Linder, E., Ruoslahti, E., and Vaheri, A., 1974, Distribution of fibroblast surface antigen, *J. Exp. Med.* **140**:1522.

Webster, H. de F., 1971, The geometry of peripheral myelin sheaths during their formation and growth in rat sciatic nerves, *J. Cell Biol.* **48**:348.

Whittaker, V. P., and Barker, L. A., 1972, The subcellular fractionation of brain tissue with special reference to the preparation of synaptosomes and their component organelles, in: *Methods of Neurochemistry,* vol. 2 (R. Fried, ed.), pp. 1–52, Marcel Dekker, New York.

Winter, J., Mirsky, R., and Kadlubowski, M., 1982, Immunocytochemical study of the appearance of P_2 in developing rat peripheral nerve: comparison with other myelin components, *J. Neurocytol.,* in press.

Wolpert, L., 1969, Positional information and the spatial pattern of differentiation, *J. Theor. Biol.* **25**:1.

Wood, P., 1976, Separation of functional Schwann cells and neurones from normal peripheral nerve tissue, *Brain Res.* **115**:361.

Yen, S.-H., and Fields, K. L., 1981, Antibodies to neurofilament, glial filament and fibroblast intermediate filament proteins bind to different cell types in the nervous system, *J. Cell Biol.* **88**:115.

7

Immunological Studies of the Retina

COLIN J. BARNSTABLE

1. INTRODUCTION

The wealth of information about the mammalian CNS that has come from anatomical and electrophysiological studies has provided many clues about the cell types, and their connections, involved in a number of neural pathways. However, neurobiologists have lacked a method for translating this information into the language of biochemistry and molecular biology so as to allow an understanding of the molecular basis of neural development and function. Antibodies provide a unique tool with which to make such a translation. They are fixable and can be coupled to enzymes, metalloproteins, fluorescent dyes, or radioactive isotopes to allow anatomical visualization of antigenic sites at the light- and electron-microscopic levels. Antibodies can be used as pharmacological agents to affect rapid physiological processes such as transmitter binding to receptors or ion channel kinetics. In addition, it may be possible to use them to study slower processes such as cellular migration and intercellular interactions. The biochemical purification of molecules can be monitored by their antigenic activity or can be achieved directly by the use of antibody affinity columns (for example, see Parham *et al.*, 1979). Similar techniques also allow the measurement of antigen me-

COLIN J. BARNSTABLE · Department of Neurobiology, Harvard Medical School, Boston, Mass. 02115.

tabolism and, in combination with other *in vitro* systems, can even allow the identification and isolation of the relevant genes (Schechter, 1974; Shapiro *et al.*, 1974).

For any one of these uses of antibodies it is important to have a monospecific antibody. In using an antibody as a link between any two approaches monospecificity becomes absolutely vital, since without it there is no longer confidence that the same antigen is being studied in the two approaches. Until recently such monospecificity could only be achieved by biochemical or genetic manipulation of the immunogen. Good examples of these approaches are the production of antisera against Thy-1, a cell surface glycoprotein found in large amounts on thymocytes and cells of the nervous system of rodents (Letarte-Muirhead *et al.*, 1975). Monospecific rabbit antisera against rat Thy-1 antigen have been prepared by injecting purified Thy-1 molecules (Barclay *et al.*, 1975). Monospecific antisera against mouse Thy-1 antigen have been prepared by cross-immunization between mouse strains bred such that the only genetic differences between them are in the Thy-1 gene (Snell and Cherry, 1972). In a few other cases the use of a biochemically pure antigen preparation has allowed the production of monospecific antisera against neural antigens. Such antisera against a phosphoprotein of synapses (Huttner and Greengard, 1979) and against myelin proteins (Lisak *et al.*, 1970) have been used successfully to study the anatomical localisation of the respective antigens (Bloom *et al.*, 1979; Mendell and Whittaker, 1978). Clearly, however, such an approach cannot be of general applicability since to unravel the molecular complexity of even a single physiological pathway would require the purification of large numbers of molecules, many of which will be present in only very small amounts.

Genetic manipulation is also of little use since without a marker for the gene(s) of interest it is impossible to monitor the breeding schedule necessary to set up the relevant congenic strains.

Thus, with these constraints it is not surprising that most of the antisera produced against nervous system antigens have been multispecific and have only begun to show any specificity after extensive absorption (Schachner, 1974; Stallcup and Cohn, 1976; Chaffee and Schachner, 1978; Brockes *et al.*, 1977). Even then some of these sera have been shown to be multispecific (Yuan *et al.*, 1977).

The approach of Köhler and Milstein (1975) by which antibody-secreting spleen cells are converted into cloned hybrid cell lines may overcome many of the problems in the immunological analysis of the nervous system. It is now possible to use heterogeneous immunogens and still derive monospecific (because they are monoclonal) antibodies (Williams *et al.*, 1977; Barnstable *et al.*, 1978; Barnstable, 1980). In theory, such antibodies could be produced against every immunogenic molecule in the nervous system. In practice, however, the range of antibodies that can be produced will be limited by the types of immunogens available as well as the sensitivity and discrimination of the assays used to detect them. The application of monoclonal antibody techniques to neurobiology is still in its infancy and the antibodies now available are more often than not due to serendipity. To produce the types of antibodies necessary to gain a full understanding of the development and function of the nervous system will require many new ways of preparing immunogens and new ways of assaying for antibodies.

In this article I would like to outline some of the approaches that have been taken in this laboratory to produce antibodies that recognize discrete cell types in the retina. In addition I would like to discuss some of the other possible approaches that will allow neuroimmunology to be what it ought to be, that is, a branch of molecular neurobiology.

2. PRODUCTION OF MONOCLONAL ANTIBODIES

2.1. Introduction

For many laboratories, the production of monoclonal antibodies has become routine. Each laboratory, however, uses its own variation of immunization, fusion, and screening protocols, and in spite of attempts to standarize the process (Fazekas de St. Groth and Scheidegger, 1980), many of the parameters for successful antibody production remain unknown. At some time in the future a rationale for the particular procedures adopted may emerge, but until then, it is still worth detailing the methods used in the preparation of any antibody.

2.2. Choice and Preparation of Immunogen

The rat retina was chosen as a source of immunogen because it was the only animal for which both a plentiful supply of adult tissue for biochemistry and a supply of neonatal material for tissue culture could readily be obtained. A microsomal fraction was prepared from retinas either immediately after dissection or after freezing in liquid N_2 and storage at $-80°C$ as outlined in Fig. 1. This preparation was chosen in preference to a tissue homogenate because it could be frozen for later use, could be given safely as intravenous injections, and represented an enrichment of about 10-fold in the cell surface markers that were the objective of this study.

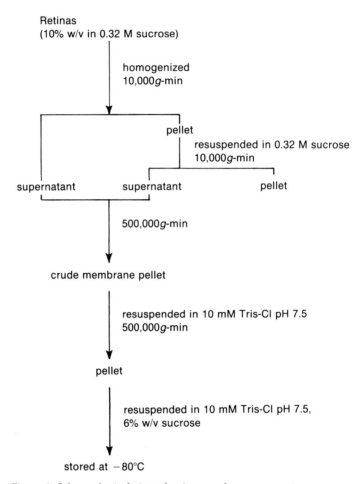

Figure 1. Scheme for isolation of retina membranes use as immunogen.

2.3. Immunization, Fusion, and Cloning

Female BALB/c mice were immunized intraperitoneally with 200 μg of retina membranes in complete Freund's adjuvant on day 0 and 200 μg of retina membranes in incomplete Freund's adjuvant on day 21. Mice were bled from the tail vein on day 42 and those making a strong response used for fusions. Fusions have been attempted with spleens from mice given only a single immunization, but the yield of hybrids and the affinity of the resulting antibodies have both been low. This reflects experience in other systems where hyperimmunization was much more efficient at eliciting high-affinity antibodies to particular portions of defined molecules (Brodsky et al., 1979). Four days before fusion, mice were injected with 100 μg of retina membranes in saline. Spleens were removed, and approximately 10^8 spleen cells were fused with 10^7 myeloma cells as described by Galfrè et al. (1977) with slight modifications. Both P3/NSI/1-Ag4-1 (Köhler and Milstein, 1975) and P3 × 63 Ag 8.653 (Kearney et al., 1979) myeloma cell lines have been used successfully. Fifty percent (w/w) polyethylene glycol (PEG) (Baker 1000) in RPMI 1640 was used as fusing agent and all manipulations were carried out at 37°C. The fusion sequence consisted of 1 ml of 50% PEG added over 1 min, after a further minute, 2 ml of serum-free RPMI 1640 were added over 2 min and then 8 ml of serum-free RPMI 1640 were added over 4 min. The fusion mixture was spun at 100g for 10 min, resuspended in RPMI 1640 + 10% FCS + 10 μg/ml gentamycin + HAT, and plated on feeder layers of secondary fibroblasts originally grown out from newborn rat lung. In successful fusions, vigorous growth has been detectable 7 days after fusion and wells have been screened for antibody production between days 10 and 14. Positive cultures were first weaned off HAT medium (Barnstable et al., 1978) and then cloned. The most successful method of cloning consisted of first plating at low density in microwells, both to enrich the positive cells in the cultures and to select for cells that grow well at low density, and then cloning cells from the most strongly positive wells in soft agar using the procedure of Cotton et al. (1973). Clones were picked from the agar, tested, recloned where necessary, and grown to larger volumes either for a source of tissue culture supernatant or to provide cells to be grown as ascites tumors in pristane-primed mice (Brodsky et al., 1979).

2.4. Binding Assays

Indirect antibody binding assays, in which the amount of antibody bound to a target is measured by the use of a suitable anti-immunoglobulin (anti-Ig) reagent, are probably the most widely used for the detection of monoclonal antibodies. They have the advantages that they can be quantitative, can be used with many different primary antibodies, and can be scaled up to permit many hundreds of samples to be assayed quickly. Generally the anti-Ig, labeled with ^{125}I or an enzyme, has been used in trace amounts [see Williams (1977) for a more detailed account of the parameters of this assay]. In the work described below, the anti-Ig was an affinity-purified rabbit anti-mouse IgG that had been pepsin-degraded and the F(ab)$'_2$ fragment isolated by gel filtration. The use of such fragments reduces the background normally encountered with whole IgG fractions or affinity-purified antibodies (Morris and Williams, 1975).

In studies of antigens or lymphocytes or cell lines (for example, Williams *et al.*, 1977; Barnstable *et al.*, 1978) it is relatively easy to prepare a uniform suspension of cells that can be used as targets for binding assays. This is not the case for a complex solid tissue such as the nervous system. Several approaches have been used to overcome this although each has its own bias. Barclay (1977) showed that it was possible to assay rabbit anti-rat brain sera on lightly homogenized and fixed rat brain. An alternative has been the use of a solid-phase assay in which membrane fragments are allowed to attach spontaneously to the wells of polyvinylchloride plates, after the assay of Segal and Klinman (1976). Such solid-phase assays have also been used successfully with detergent-solubilized membranes (for example, see Carlson and Kelly, 1980). Solid-phase assays are somewhat variable in that some membranes and membrane components attach to plastic surfaces much better than others. In a characterized system this can be advantageous, but it can be a disadvantage in a general screening assay for a variety of antibodies.

The antibodies discussed in this chapter were detected by screening culture supernatants on fixed-retina homogenates. A 10% suspension of retina was lightly homogenized and fixed for 30 min in 0.5% paraformaldehyde in 0.1 M phosphate buffer pH 7.4. After extensive washing in 5% BSA in PBS the 10,000g-min pellet was resuspended in wash buffer and frozen at −80°C. for the assay, homogenate was diluted in 5% BSA in PBS and 25 µl of this suspension was incubated with 25 µl of culture supernatant for 1 hr at room temperature. After washing three times with 0.1% BSA in PBS the pellet was resuspended in 50 µl of ^{125}I-labeled anti-mouse IgG. After incubation for 1 hr at room temperature and washing as before, bound radioactivity was determined in a gamma counter. Some, but not all, antibodies detected in this assay could also be detected using a solid-phase assay in which the immunizing membrane preparation was allowed to attach to polyvinylchloride plates.

2.5. *Immunocytochemistry*

Screening for antibodies by indirect immunofluorescent or immunoperoxidase labeling of tissue sections has the disadvantage of being less quantitative than the above binding assays but has the advantage of providing information as to the cellular or subcellular localization of the antigen. Indeed, this assay may be the only one possible when screening for antibodies that recognize molecules present on only a very small proportion of the cells of that tissue. Such an assay has been used to screen for antibodies recognizing cell types of the leech nervous system (Zipser and McKay, 1981) and frog neuromuscular synapses (Burden, 1981).

The antibodies against retina cells described below were first detected by an indirect radioactive binding assay and only later assayed using immunofluorescence. For this, rats were generally perfused through the left ventricle with 1% paraformaldehyde, 0.1% glutaraldehyde in 0.1 M sodium phosphate buffer pH 7.6. For retinas, but not other brain regions, adequate tissue preservation was also achieved by rapid dissection and immersion fixation. After fixation for 1 hr at 4°C, tissue was soaked in 30% (w/v) sucrose overnight at 4°C. Sections (10–20 μm) were cut on a freezing microtome and dried onto subbed slides. Sections were preincubated with 5% BSA in phosphate buffer for 1 hr at 4°C and then with primary antibody for 18 hr at 4°C. The slides were washed with two changes of a large excess of phosphate buffer for 10 min each at 4°C, and the sections were then treated with a Rhodamine-conjugated goat anti-mouse IgG (Cappell) diluted in a solution of equal parts of 5% BSA in phosphate buffer and normal rabbit serum. Before use, the rabbit serum was passed over a column of mouse IgG coupled to Sepharose 4B to remove any heterophile anti-mouse IgG antibodies. After incubation for 45 min at room temperature the slides were again washed with two changes of phosphate buffer and then coverslipped using 50% glycerol in phosphate buffer as mounting medium. Slides were examined with a Zeiss IM35 microscope. Fluorescence photographs were taken using epi-illumination on H&W Control film with a 2 min exposure.

For electron microscopy retinas were dissected and fixed in 2% glutaraldehyde, 2% paraformaldehyde in 0.12 M phosphate buffer pH 7.3 for 1 hr at 4°C. Retinas were embedded in gelatin–albumin polymerized with glutaraldehyde and vibratome sectioned at 100 μm (Fekete and Barnstable, 1981). Sections were stored in phosphate buffer containing 8% dextrose and 0.2 mM $CaCl_2$. Sections were washed for 30 min each in 20 mM NH_4Cl in PBS and 1% BSA, 1% goat serum, 0.05% Triton X-100 in PBS. All subsequent antibody dilutions were made in the latter buffer. Sections were incubated in primary antibody overnight at 4°C. After six rinses in PBS over 1 hr, sections were treated with either ferritin-conjugated goat anti-mouse IgG (Cappell) for 1 hr at room temperature or a goat anti-mouse IgG antibody (Miles) as a linker for a peroxidase–antiperoxidase (PAP) complex. After extensive washing the latter sections were treated with a mouse PAP complex (Sternberger–Meyer) for 1 hr at room temperature; after further washing, the peroxidase was reacted with diaminobenzidine.

Both ferritin- and peroxidase-labeled tissue sections were treated with 2% OsO_4 in phosphate buffer + 7% dextrose and traces of $CaCl_2$ for 2 hr. After washing tissue was stained en bloc with 2% uranyl acetate, washed, dehydrated through alcohols and propylene oxide, and embedded in Epon 812. Thin sections were mounted on grids and stained for 90 sec each with uranyl acetate and lead citrate.

3. MONOCLONAL ANTIBODIES THAT LABEL PHOTORECEPTORS

3.1. Labeling of Adult Tissue

Three classes of antibody have been found that specifically label photoreceptors. Their patterns of labeling of sections of adult rat retinas are shown in Fig. 2. The first class of antibody, exemplified by RET-P1 (Fig. 2a, b), labeled the whole photoreceptor layer with the exception of the outer plexiform layer. A clear ring of fluorescence was found around almost all of the photoreceptor cell bodies. The packing between the cell bodies appeared looser toward the outer limiting membrane, and the intervening spaces often showed fluorescence. This was probably due to the fibers which connect the cell bodies with their inner segments. The photoreceptor inner segments were labeled at about the same intensity as the cell bodies, but the outer segments had a much brighter fluorescence. These differences presumably represented differences in antigen density, which supports previous observations that the composition of the outer segment membrane is different from that of the rest of the cell (Young, 1968; Papermaster et al., 1978).

Very different patterns of labeling of photoreceptors were given by the other classes of antibody exemplified by RET-P2 (Fig. 2c, d) and RET-P3 (Fig. 2e, f). RET-P2 labeled the outer segments; the inner segments and cell bodies were unlabeled as far as could be judged in the fluorescence assay. RET-P3, on the other hand, labeled only the cell bodies.

The rat retina consists almost entirely of rods (La Vail, 1976), so that judging whether or not RET-P1, RET-P2, or RET-P3 reacted with both rods and cones was impossible. To investigate this, a number of different species were examined to see whether the antibodies reacted with a retina containing a higher proportion of cones. To date RET-P1 has reacted with all species tested, including goldfish, salamander, turtle, mouse, rabbit, and rat. RET-P1 is an autoantibody since it reacted with photoreceptors of BALB/c mice from which the antibody-producing

OS
IS
OLM
ONL
OPL
INL
IPL
GCL

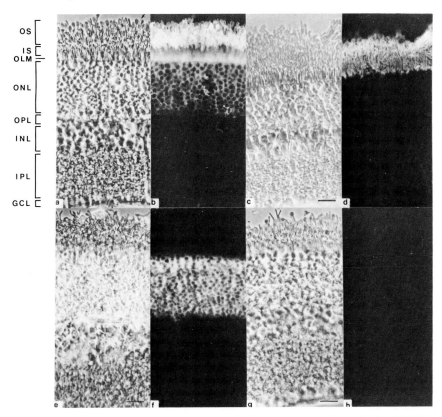

Figure 2. Immunofluorescent labeling of sections of adult rat retina by antibodies RET-P1, RET-P2, and RET-P3. (a, b) RET-P1 antibody showing reaction with the photoreceptor layer. (c, d) RET-P2 antibody showing reaction with photoreceptor outer segments. (e, f) RET-P3 antibody showing reaction with photoreceptor cell bodies. (g, h) Control using a monoclonal antibody against a human cell surface glycoprotein. (a, c, e, g) Phase contrast; (b, d, f, h) fluorescence. OS, outer segments; IS, inner segments; OLM, outer limiting membrane; ONL, outer nuclear layer; OPL, outer plexiform layer; INL, inner nuclear layer; IPL, inner plexiform layer; GCL, ganglion cell layer. Scale bar represents 20 μm. (From Barnstable, 1980.)

spleen cell was derived. Both RET-P2 and RET-P3 antigenic determinants, on the other hand, seem to be restricted to rat. A group of photoreceptors in a section of retina from the tiger salamander (*Ambystoma tigrinum*) is shown in Fig. 3. Cells 1, 3, and 5 are rods, although the outer segment of cell 3 was removed during dissection. When treated with RET-P1 all three cells were labeled throughout their length, with the most intense fluorescence being in the outer segment. The bright

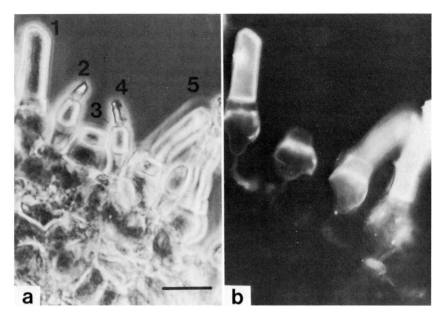

Figure 3. Immunofluorescent labeling of tiger salamander photoreceptors by antibody RET-P1. (a) Phase contrast; (b) fluorescence. Cells 1, 3, and 5 are rods; cells 2 and 6 are cones. Scale bar represents 20 μm. (From Barnstable, 1980.)

band(s) at the junction of the inner and outer segments was probably due to labeling of the deep membrane folds at this region. These represent the initial stage of pinching off of the disks of the outer segment (Cohen, 1970), which might suggest that RET-P1 is also present in the disks (see below). Cells 2 and 4 have the morphology of cones, that is, narrower cell bodies, narrower but longer inner segments, and slender outer segments. The outer segments of cells 2 and 4 are almost certainly damaged, but there is no trace of fluorescence on any part of the cells. This would indicate that, in salamanders at least, RET-P1 is restricted to rods. RET-P1 also labels rods but not cones in goldfish (unpublished experiments in collaboration with P. Johns). As can also be seen in Fig. 3, the axons and synaptic pedicles of the rods were labeled. In several cases fine labeled processes were found to be given off from the thick pedicles. The lack of labeling of the outer plexiform layer in rat retina shown in Fig. 2a may thus be simply because such labeling was below the threshold for visualization or alternatively may be real and may represent a difference in antigen compartmentalization between the two species.

Further evidence for the subcellular distribution of RET-P1 antigen in rat photoreceptors was obtained by labeling tissue using the PAP method (Sternberger, 1979) and examining it in the electron microscope. Figure 4 (a,c) shows that virtually no nonspecific labeling occurred with the reagents used. Figure 4 (b, d) also shows that both inner and outer segments were labeled around their plasma membranes. In the outer segments, however, two areas of labeling were evident (Fig. 4d). The first was, as expected, around the plasma membrane. The second was on the ends of the photoreceptor disks.

It was not clear whether this represented diffusion of peroxidase reaction product from the plasma membrane or incomplete penetration of the PAP complexes into the photoreceptor disks. With ferritin-labeling the situation was much clearer. Once again, clear specific labeling of the outer face of the outer segment plasma membrane could be seen (Fig. 5a, b). No ferritin labeling could be seen in regions of intact disks, but clear labeling of the inner face of the disks was observed at points where the outer segments were broken open (Fig. 5c). In sections showing the base of the outer segment and the connecting cilium (Fig. 5d) labeling was observed in the membrane folds that had not yet pinched off completely to form disks. Ferritin labeling was also apparent on the inner segment membrane but, in accordance with the fluorescence results, was at a lower density than on the outer segment membrane. Thus it seems quite clear that RET-P1 is a photoreceptor membrane molecule that in the outer segment is on both the outer face of the plasma membrane and the internal face of the disk membrane. There is some indication that the same is not true of RET-P2. When retina membranes are prepared under isotonic conditions a certain specific activity of RET-P1 and RET-P2 antigens can be defined (Table I). Upon solubilization with either NP-40 or sodium deoxycholate (Na DoC), or upon heating the membranes, the measured amount of RET-P1 greatly increases, whereas that of RET-P2 antigen remains constant. Since RET-P1 antigen seems to be present on the inner face of the disks, the most likely explanation of these results is that detergents or heating open up the sealed disks and make much more RET-P1 antigen available for antibody binding. Since RET-P2 antigen does not change its specific activity upon detergent or heat treatment it is probably not within the disks. If this is the case then it suggests that only a portion of the outer segment membrane gets incorporated into disks. The mechanisms by which such segregation could occur is not known.

The three antibodies described above almost certainly recognize previously undescribed antigens of photoreceptors. An antigen, termed S antigen, has been described that is distributed on photoreceptors in

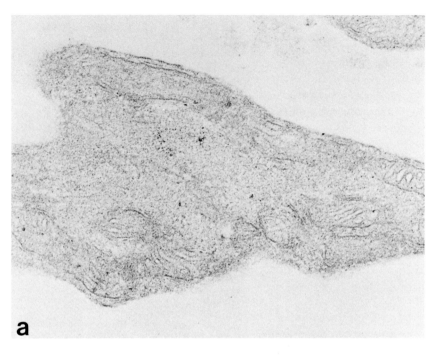

a

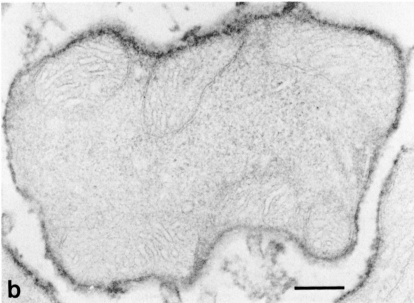

b

Figure 4. Labeling of adult rat photoreceptors by antibody RET-P1 using PAP. (a) Control, inner segment; (b) RET-P1, inner segment; (c) Control, outer segment; (d) RET-P1, outer segment. The controls were taken through all incubations with buffer substituted for RET-P1. Even though detergent was present in all buffers, the plasma membrane shows uninterrupted segments and the general tissue preservation is good. Peroxidase reaction

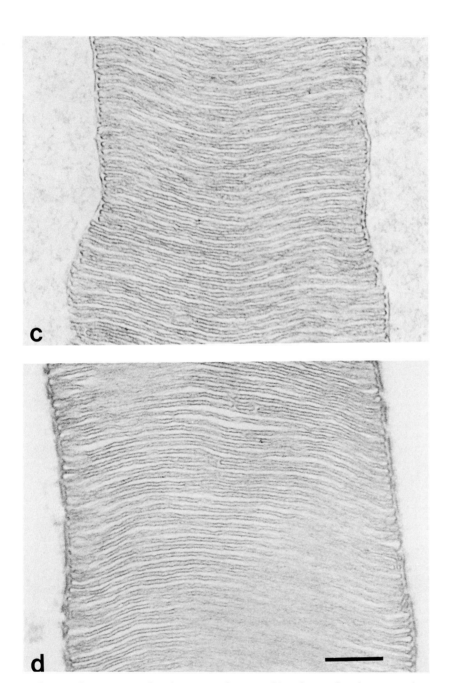

product can be seen over the plasma membrane in (b) and over the plasma membrane and the outer edges of the disks in (d). Any differences in intensity between (b) and (d) are more a reflection of depth in the tissue section than differences in antigen density. Scale bar represents 250 nm. (From Fekete and Barnstable, 1981).

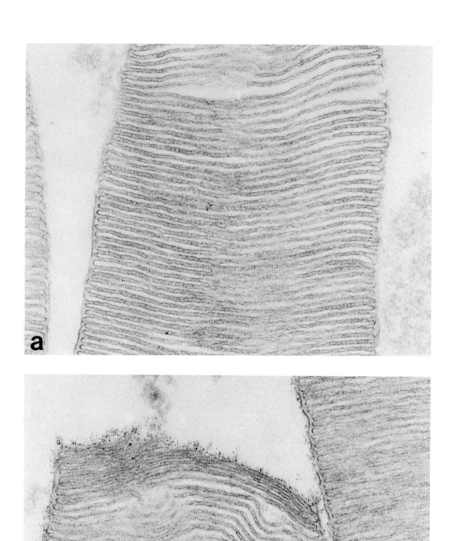

Figure 5. Labeling of adult rat photoreceptors by antibody RET-P1 using ferritin-conjugated second antibody. (a) Control outer segment with buffer substituted for RET-P1. (b) Outer segments showing ferritin grains outside the plasma membranes. In (a) and (b) the interior of the outer segments can be seen as a series of alternating light and dark bands. At the edges of the disks it is clear that the light bands correspond to the space inside the disks and the dark bands to the cytoplasmic space between disks. Following these bands to the

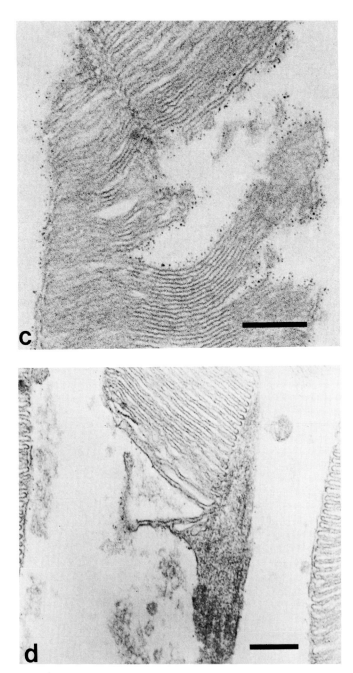

broken edge of the outer segment in (b), it is clear that the ferritin grains are adjacent to an inside face of a disk. Similarly, the broken outer segment shown in (c) shows ferritin labeling only on inner faces of disks. In (d) the base of an outer segment is shown with its connecting cilium. Ferritin grains can be seen on the membrane that has invaginated prior to forming a disk. Scale bars represent 250 nm for (a) and (b) and 200 nm for (c) and (d). (From Fekete and Barnstable, 1981.)

Table I. Subcellular Distribution of RET-P1 and RET-P2 Antigens

Fraction	RET P1		RET P2	
	ID_{50}^a (U/mg)	% Recovery	ID_{50}^a (U/mg)	% Recovery
Homogenate	43.5	100	1000	100
Nuclear pellet	4.4	2.1	111	1.3
Low-speed S''	34.5	38.7	1428	88.7
Cytosol	4.0	15.3	80	3.9
High-speed pellet	71.4	52.1	5882	100
NP-40 S''	279,417	106,192	5461	68.4
DoC S''	80,333	46,406	4779	66.3
100°C, 10 min	63,467	—	6497	—

[a] The specific activity is given as ID_{50} units per milligram of protein. These units are calculated from the amount of a particular fraction needed to inhibit a standard binding assay by 50%. Recoveries are calculated from the total number of ID_{50} units present in a given fraction.

a similar way to RET-P1 antigen (Wacker *et al.*, 1977). S antigen is thought to be one of the major antigenic stimuli in the autoimmune disease experimental allergic uveitis. It is a soluble protein with an apparent molecular mass of 50,000 daltons and is not present in developing retina. Both of these properties distinguish it from RET-P1 (see Table I and Section 3.2). The other well-characterized photoreceptor molecule is the visual pigment molecule rhodopsin. A rabbit antiserum raised against bovine rhodopsin labeled both outer and inner segments of frog photoreceptors (Dewey *et al.*, 1969). A monoclonal antibody against rhodopsin (a gift of M. Applebury) gave a similar pattern of labeling in rat retina. This pattern was clearly different from that of RET-P1, RET-P2, and RET-P3. In addition, none of these antibodies was inhibited by a partially purified preparation of bovine rhodopsin (a gift of E. Schwartz), and as described below, the developmental time of appearance of rhodopsin differs from that of each of the three antibodies described here.

3.2. Developmental Expression of Photoreceptor Antigens

To determine the time at which each antigen appeared during development, retinas were fixed and sectioned at various postnatal ages. RET-P1 was the only antibody found to react on postnatal day 1. Figure 6 shows the labeling pattern given by this antibody. (The section shown is from a day 2 retina, by which time more cells are labeled so that more than one positive cell per field could be shown). The labeled cells do

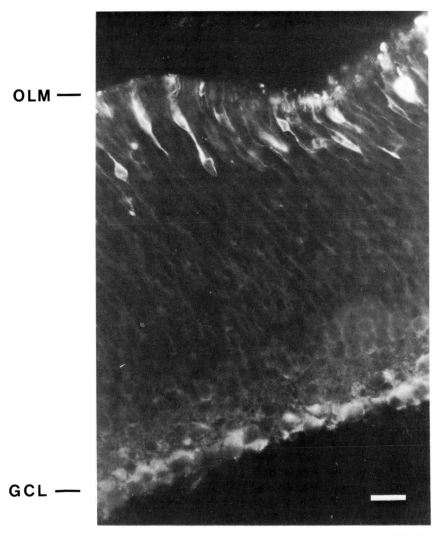

OLM —

GCL —

Figure 6. Immunofluorescent labeling of 2-day postnatal rat retina by antibody RET-P1. A small proportion of cells at the ventricular margin show specific fluorescence. This fluorescence was relatively weak and required a longer photographic exposure which has resulted in the tissue background fluorescence becoming visible. Scale bar represents 20 μm. (From Barnstable, 1981.)

not resemble adult photoreceptors but are elongated bipolar cells. One of the two fine processes given off from the cell bodies was directed vitreally and seemed to end toward the middle of the retina. The other process ended at the ventricular surface in a small, brightly labeled structure which presumably corresponded to the primary cilium from which point the photoreceptor outer segments grow (Nilsson, 1964). Thus the morphology of these labeled cells closely matches that pre- dicted for developing photoreceptors on the basis of serial EM recon- structions of embryonic mouse retinas (J. W. Hinds and P. L. Hinds, 1979). The number of labeled cells in the outer portion of the retina increased with time until essentially all were RET-P1 positive on about day 6. Since the first labeled cells were found in all areas of the retina, it seems unlikely that expression of RET-P1 antigen is induced by any diffusible factor acting upon an equally competent cell population. Per- haps more likely is that the timing of RET-P1 antigen expression is related to an event such as final mitosis of photoreceptor precursors.

By day 8, photoreceptor outer segments are forming and the outer plexiform layer is present (Fig. 7a). All the cells in the now discernible outer nuclear layer are RET-P1 positive (Fig. 7b). The outer segments are labeled, but the outer plexiform layer is unlabeled, as is the case in the adult. Some RET-P1-positive cells can be seen in the inner nuclear layer. These do not seem to be a sectioning artifact, since they have been found at various focal depths in the sections. They have also been found in both central and peripheral areas of the retina. It is not known whether these cells migrate up through the outer plexiform layer and become normal photoreceptors or die because of their aberrant position.

The visual pigment molecule, rhodopsin, was detectable at days 5–6, the time of outer segment formation and first appeared as a series of brightly fluorescent spots at the outer limiting membrane (Fig. 8).

RET-P2 antigen was also first present on days 5–6 and also appeared as a series of bright spots at the outer limiting membrane. As far as could be judged, these spots corresponded to the initial outgrowths from the primary cilia. It is interesting to note that both rhodopsin and RET-P2 were restricted to the outer segment region from their first appearance. Thus, whatever the mechanism of restriction of antigen mobility, it is operative at or before the time of outer segment formation. In many series of animals examined, both rhodopsin and RET-P2 ap- peared at the same time, that is, day 5 or 6. Occasionally, however, an animal was found that expressed RET-P2 but not rhodopsin, suggesting a small difference in their times of expression.

RET-P3 was not detectable until days 12–13, just before the time of eye opening. At its first appearance the morphology of the retina was

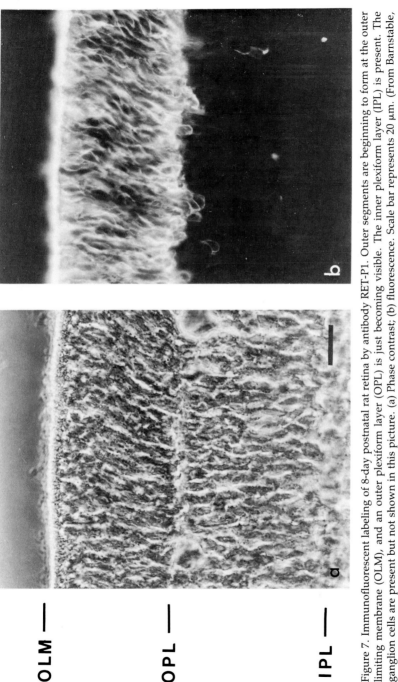

OLM —

OPL —

IPL —

Figure 7. Immunofluorescent labeling of 8-day postnatal rat retina by antibody RET-P1. Outer segments are beginning to form at the outer limiting membrane (OLM), and an outer plexiform layer (OPL) is just becoming visible. The inner plexiform layer (IPL) is present. The ganglion cells are present but not shown in this picture. (a) Phase contrast; (b) fluorescence. Scale bar represents 20 μm. (From Barnstable, 1981.)

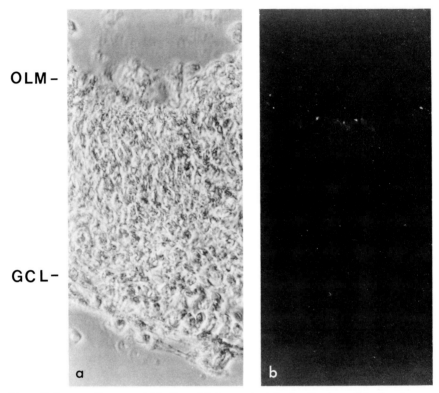

Figure 8. Immunofluorescent labeling of 6-day postnatal rat retina by antirhodopsin antibody. The only detectable fluorescence is the row of bright spots at the outer limiting membrane. See Fig. 2 caption for key. Scale bar represents 20 μm. (From Barnstable, 1981.)

essentially that of the adult and the labeling pattern given by RET-P3 antibody was indistinguishable from that previously shown (Fig. 2e, f).

Three phases of photoreceptor development have been detected by the antibodies RET-P1, RET-P2, and RET-P3. The first phase occurs during or shortly after commitment of precursor cells to become photoreceptors and is marked by the appearance of RET-P1 antigen. RET-P2 antigen (and rhodopsin) marks the series of molecular changes that occur as photoreceptor inner and outer segments form. The appearance of RET-P3 antigen marks a phase of cell maturation during which photoreceptors become capable of generating electrical responses to light. Of course, other antibodies may detect molecules appearing at intermediate times, and it may become necessary to think of photoreceptor development as a continuum of molecular events rather than discrete phases.

4. MONOCLONAL ANTIBODIES THAT LABEL MÜLLER CELLS

Except for a few astrocytic cells in the optic fiber layer, Müller cells are the only glial cell type in the retina. They have a unique morphology in that they are the only cell type to extend radially across the retina from the outer limiting membrane to the inner limiting membrane (Miller and Dowling, 1970; Uga and Smelser, 1973a,b). The essential features of their structure as shown in the Golgi-stained cell in Fig. 9a were clearly picked out in the immunofluorescent labeling of sections of adult

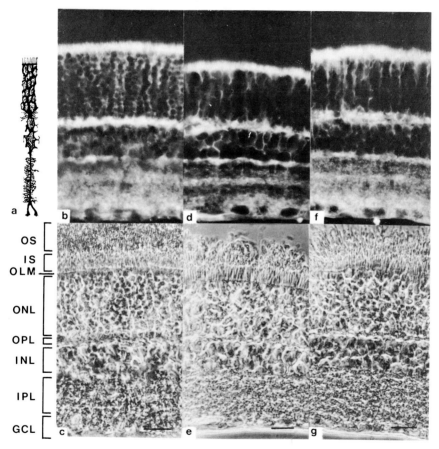

Figure 9. Immunofluorescent labeling of sections of adult rat retina by antibodies RET-G1, RET-G2, and RET-G3. (a) Müller cell from a Golgi-impregnated retina as drawn by S. R. Cajal (Cajal, 1972). (b, c) RET-G1 antibody; (d, e) RET-G2 antibody; (f, g) RET-G3 antibody. (b, d, f) Fluorescence; (c, e, g) phase contrast. Designation of retinal layers is described in Fig. 2 caption. Scale bar represents 20 μm. (From Barnstable, 1980.)

rat retina given by antibodies RET-G1 (Fig. 9b, c), RET-G2 (Fig. 9d, e), and RET-G3 (Fig. 9f, g). At the outer limiting membrane each antibody labeled the fine, fingerlike Müller cell processes that extend up between the inner half of the photoreceptor inner segments. Thick radial processes passing through the outer nuclear layer were also labeled, although the single focal plane shown in the photographs was not always adequate to show a single process traversing the whole width of that layer. Virtually no rings of fluorescence could be seen around the photoreceptor cell bodies, indicating that they had not reacted with the antibodies. The labeling in the inner nuclear layer was harder to interpret but probably represented Müller fibers following the contours of the cell bodies in this region on their way to the inner plexiform layer.

In very few cases was it possible to see a clear ring of fluorescence around a cell body as would have been expected if the neurons of the inner nuclear layer had been labeled. Those few cell bodies that seemed to be labeled had the position expected for Müller cell bodies. The radial Müller fibers give off fine tangential processes in both plexiform layers, and these were labeled by all three antibodies shown in Fig. 9. The labeling of the inner plexiform layer showed three bands of higher intensity. One band was located at the junction of the inner nuclear and inner plexiform layers, one band was about halfway through the inner plexiform layer, and the third thick band was at the junction of the inner plexiform and ganglion cell layers and was continuous with the labeling of the bulbous feet that surround the ganglion cell bodies and optic fibers and end at the inner limiting membrane. This banded appearance of the inner plexiform layer was very similar to the autoradiographic labeling of Müller cells seen following uptake of radioactive GABA *in vitro* (Fig. 10) (unpublished experiment in collaboration with R. W. Baughman). The increased labeling presumably reflects an increased density of tangential glial projections in those sublaminae of the plexiform layer. An almost reciprocal pattern of labeling of the inner plexiform layer was given by a monoclonal anti-rat Thy-1 antibody (a gift from A. Williams). Thy-1 is reported to be a neuron-specific marker (Raff *et al.*, 1979), although its presence on different cell types in the intact nervous system has not been unambiguously assigned (Barclay, 1979). The ways in which these lamination patterns are correlated with particular structures of defined cell types will require histological analysis at higher levels of resolution.

As a further demonstration that antibody RET-G1 was reacting with Müller cells, immunofluorescent labeling of enzymatically dissociated adult rat retina cells was carried out. The results (Fig. 11) clearly show that this antibody labeled cells with the morphology characteristic of

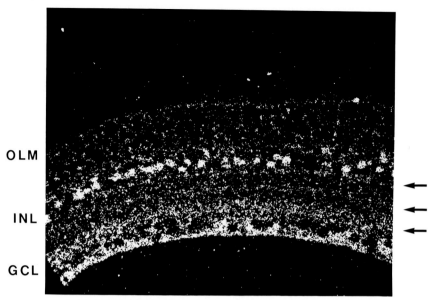

OLM

INL

GCL

Figure 10. Darkfield autoradiograph of a section of adult rat retina after [³H]GABA uptake *in vitro*. Pieces of retina were incubated with 1 μm [³H]GABA, rinsed, fixed, and processed for autoradiography. The retinal layers are as described in Fig. 2 caption. The three arrows to the right of the figure show the bands of increased grain density running through the inner plexiform layer. (R. W. Baughman and C. J. Barnstable, unpublished results.)

Müller cells. A variety of other neuronal cells and unidentifiable cell bodies were not labeled in these preparations.

RET-G1, RET-G2, and RET-G3 react with different determinants, and probably different molecules, of Müller cells. The strongest evidence for this comes from the finding that they are detectable at different stages of retina development. RET-G1 is present at birth, but RET-G2 is only detectable at days 6–7. Although in the adult these two antibodies show a very similar pattern of labeling, in young rats there was a clear difference. As shown in Fig. 12a, RET-G1 labeled the inner plexiform layer more heavily than the inner nuclear layer in postnatal day 8 rat retina. RET-G2, on the other hand, labeled the inner nuclear layer more heavily (Fig. 12b). RET-G3 was detectable only on days 12–13, shortly before the time of eye opening.

Further evidence for the differences between RET-G1 and RET-G2 or RET-G3 has been obtained by absorption analysis. All three antibodies could be absorbed by retina membrane, but only RET-G1 could be absorbed by membranes from cerebral cortex or cerebellum (Barnstable, 1980). Another three antibodies that label the Müller cells, RET-G4, RET-

G5, and RET-G6 were absorbed by retina membrane but not other membrane. These results indicate both that Müller cells have a number of molecular determinants which distinguish them from glia elsewhere in the CNS and that they have some determinants in common. It is known that Müller cells share certain properties with astrocytes elsewhere in the CNS. These include GABA uptake (Iversen and Kelly, 1975), K^+-ion transport (Kuffler *et al.*, 1966), and close apposition to neuronal processes (Peters *et al.*, 1976). Whether RET-G1 is involved in any of these functions is not yet clear. It is harder to envisage what the Müller-cell-specific determinants could be. A trivial explanation would be that they represent isotypic variants of molecules carrying out common functions. More intriguing is the possibility that Müller cells play an active role in retina development. The expression of different Müller cell membrane molecules at different times during development and to some extent on different regions of the cell (cf. Fig. 12) might be an influence on the migration and/or differentiation of adjacent neuronal cells.

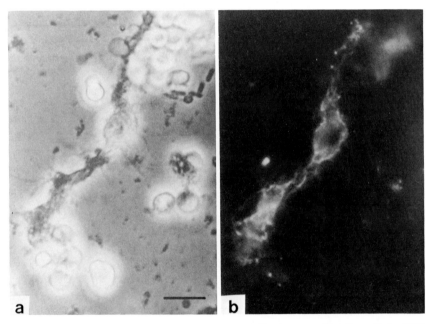

Figure 11. Immunofluorescent labeling of enzymatically dissociated Müller cells by RET-G1 antibody. Retinas were dissected from adult rats and cells dissociated by the method of Sarthy and Lam (1979). The cell suspension was allowed to settle to the bottom of Petri dishes and the labeling carried out as usual, with care being taken not to disturb the cells during the buffer rinses. Scale bar represents 10 µm. (From Barnstable, 1980.)

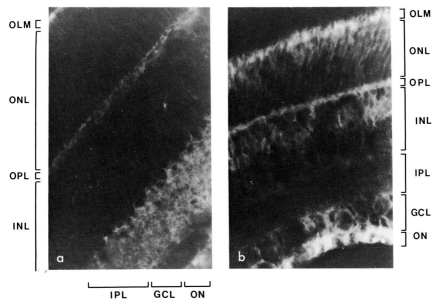

Figure 12. Immunofluorescent labeling of sections of 8-day-postnatal rat retina by antibodies RET-G1 and RET-G2. (a) Labeling by RET-G1 showing the greatest intensity over the inner plexiform layer. (b) Labeling by RET-G2 showing greatest intensity over the inner nuclear layer and ganglion cell layer with little labeling over the inner plexiform layer. See Fig. 2 caption for key. Scale bar represents 20 μm. (From Barnstable, 1981.)

5. DISCUSSION

One of the first advantages of antibodies that was listed in the introduction was the ability to use antibodies in light- and electron-microscopic studies. To be useful for this, however, the antibodies should react with only restricted subpopulations or restricted regions of neural cells. The results given above clearly show that it is possible to produce antibodies of this type. Antibodies RET-P1, RET-P2, and RET-P3 recognize only a single cell type, photoreceptors, in the rat CNS. As well as raising a number of intriguing questions about the formation and maintenance of different membrane compartments within the cells, these antibodies have a variety of other uses. The first, and the one explored above, is their use as probes of photoreceptor development. Having defined a normal pattern of development in terms of times of antigen expression, it is now possible to design experiments to test the influence of extrinsic factors upon this pattern. Such factors might include steroids, which have been shown to cause precocious expression of a glial-specific enzyme in retina (Moscona and Piddington, 1966), pigment epithelium, or a variety of other local and distant neural influences. The advantage of using antibodies in such a study is that it will be possible to study discrete molecular events in development rather than more complex functional or morphological development.

Another use of these antiphotoreceptor antibodies will be in the preparation and study of isolated photoreceptors. Since RET-P1 is expressed on the cell surface of photoreceptors early in retina development, when cells can be readily dissociated, it can be used to isolate cells by means of a fluorescence activated cell sorter or by any of several other affinity techniques. Such purified cell populations can then be used for a wide variety of biochemical and developmental studies, not least of which might be an analysis to determine the nature of the chemical transmitter used by photoreceptors.

These antibodies will also be helpful in resolving a long-standing debate about the relationship of certain pineal cells to retina photoreceptors. Pinealocytes of various submammalian vertebrates have several morphological features in common with retinal photoreceptors (Eakin and Westfall, 1959; van de Kamer, 1965). In rats such similarities are only observed during the first 2–3 weeks of life (Zimmerman and Tso, 1975). By analyzing antibody labeling of pineal tissue of neonatal rats, as well as of lower vertebrates, it may be possible to establish molecular similarities between the two cell types.

Six antibodies that react specifically with Müller cells in the adult rat retina have been analyzed. These also indicate that cell-type-specific antibodies can be produced using impure immunogens. Since only one of them, RET-G1, labeled glial cells elsewhere in the rat CNS, the results suggest that the greater resolving power of monoclonal antibodies may well reveal many related subclasses among what had previously been thought of as a single cell type.

The antibodies described in this article have recognized the two major subclasses of retinal cells, namely, photoreceptors and Müller cells. These types of antibody have been the easiest to produce, both because of the proportion of their membranes in the immunogen and because the target particles used in the screening assay probably selected for their detection. Using the methods described in Section 2, a number of antibodies that recognize most neurons, but not Müller cells, in retina have been produced, although none has been selective for any neuronal subclasses. By using a different combination of immunogen and screening assays we have recently produced an antibody that, in retina, appears to react only with ganglion cells (manuscript in preparation). Thus it seems likely that it will be possible to produce antibodies that mark each cell type in a given region of the CNS. This conclusion has recently been strengthened by results from an invertebrate system.

In studies of the leech nervous system, antibodies were produced that labeled only a single pair of cells in each midbody ganglion (Zipser and McKay, 1981). Other antibodies were found that labeled groups of cells that shared a common function, for example, pressure-sensitive cells. It is not clear whether these antibodies were detecting common features such as neurotransmitter systems or were detecting "network" molecules signaling the functional relatedness of the cells. Their production, however, does indicate the degree of specificity that can be obtained with monoclonal antibodies.

The cell-type-specific antibodies discussed in this article are only one way in which immunological methods can be of use in neurobiological studies. Of great importance will be antibodies that recognize functional components of neural systems such as enzymes, receptors, ion channels, and most particularly those molecules responsible for the formation and maintenance of synapses. Most of the available immunogens and most assay systems currently being used are, however, unlikely to detect such molecules. Most membrane, synaptosome, or synaptic fractions have such a low specific activity of any one of those components that there will be insufficient material to elicit an immune response without giving unrealistically large doses of immunogen. Even if a response is generated, then very large numbers of hybrids will have to be screened to detect the relevant antibody. Again, most assays using homogenates, membranes, or reactions on tissue sections will probably fail because of specific activity or threshold problems, or both.

There are however, ways to overcome these problems. For the immunogen there are a number of possibilities. The first is a crude biochemical fractionation. By taking glycoproteins, glycolipids, or even a more purified material as immunogen, certain components will be enriched by as much as 100-fold. More satisfactory would be specific purification schemes. These can be designed where there is an independent assay to monitor purification, for example, ligand-binding to receptors or inhibition of cell interactions (Rutishauser et al., 1978). An alternative is the use of cell lines expressing the property of interest. Many of the neuroblastomas and mutagen-induced neural cell lines currently available seem to represent immature cells and do not express high levels of transmitter synthesizing enzymes or form synapses (Schubert et al., 1974; Kidokoro et al., 1975). Somatic cell hybrids between these and defined primary neuronal cells might be one way to make such cell lines more generally useful (Minna et al., 1972; Chalazonitis et al., 1975; Trisler et al., 1979).

For the assays, perhaps the greatest progress will come when they are designed not to measure how much antibody binds to a particular target but rather the effect that antibody has upon defined physiological functions of a target. Such assays might include effects upon neurite outgrowth and fasciculation, blocking or modulation of specific classes of synapse formation, changes in transmitter release or effect, and changes in specific ion channel behavior as monitored by electrophysiological measurements of ion conductances.

The development of these assays is only just beginning and many questions have yet to be resolved. For example, how do cells respond to antibody binding to their surfaces? Are there general changes in membrane turnover that could give spurious results? What proportion of antigenic sites must be occupied to see an effect? That is, is there a threshold for an all-or-none effect or will there be a graded response? In addition, the kinetic aspects of antibody application and washout have yet to be fully resolved for assays involving electrophysiological recordings.

Related to the topic of assays is the problem of adequate anatomical localization of antigen which was touched upon in Section 3. Many antigens are sensitive to fixation, yet without adequate fixation, tissue preservation is generally not good enough to allow electron-microscopic localization of antibody binding. The other aspect of this is the problem of antibody penetration into tissue. Even in the presence of 0.05% Triton X-100 there was poor penetration of RET-P1 into photoreceptor disks. Similar problems will almost certainly arise for antigens present in dense areas of neuropil. Resolution of these problems must take place before antibodies can be regarded as truly useful anatomical tools.

As all these techniques become refined, neuroimmunology will take its place as one of the very powerful techniques available to neurobiologists. The cause for excitement in this is that the membrane resistances, capacitances, and pumps beloved of biophysicists; the intramembraneous particles of anatomists; and the recognition "lock-and-key" molecules of developmental biologists can all be named, isolated, and studied as real molecules. Perhaps immunological methods will also answer the most fundamental question in neurobiology, the mechanism by which nerve terminals recognize and interact with their correct target cells. Over 30 years ago Sperry postulated a mechanism of chemoaffinity to explain neuronal interactions (Sperry, 1950), but there is little firm biochemical evidence for or against this postulate and so the existence of such mechanisms remains an open question. With the increasing pace of change that monoclonal antibodies are bringing to biology, we may have only a short time to wait for an answer.

ACKNOWLEDGMENTS

I should like to thank Torsten Wiesel for his continuing encouragement and support, and members of the Harvard Neurobiology Department for help and advice. The work from this laboratory described in this article was supported by grants EY00606 (to Torsten Wiesel), EY01995 and EY03735 from the NIH, as well as fellowship DRG-242 from the Damon Runyon–Walter Winchell Cancer Fund.

6. REFERENCES

Barclay, A. N., 1977, A radioimmunoassay to recognise new brain differentiation antigens, *Brain Res.* **133**:139.

Barclay, A. N., 1979, Localization of the Thy-1 antigen in the cerebellar cortex of rat brain by immunofluorescence during postnatal development, *J. Neurochem.* **32**:1249.

Barclay, A. N., Letarte-Muirhead, M., and Williams, A. F., 1975, Purification of the Thy-1 molecule from rat brain, *Biochem. J.* **151**:699.

Barnstable, C. J., 1980, Monoclonal antibodies which recognise different cell types in the rat retina, *Nature (London)* **286**:231.

Barnstable, C. J., 1981, Developmental studies of the rat retina using monoclonal antibodies, in: *Monoclonal Antibodies to Neural Antigens* (R. McKay, M. C. Raff, and L. F. Reichardt, eds.), p. 219, Cold Spring Harbor Press, Cold Spring Harbor.

Barnstable, C. J., Bodmer, W. F., Brown, G., Galfré, G., Milstein, C., Williams, A. F., and Ziegler, A., 1978, Production of monoclonal antibodies to group A erythrocytes, HLA and other human cell surface antigens—New tools for genetic analysis, *Cell* **14**:9.

Bloom, F. E., Veda, T., Battenberg, E., and Greengard, P., 1979, Immunocytochemical localization, in synapses, of protein I, an endogenous substrate for protein kinases in mammalian brain, *Proc. Natl. Acad. Sci. U.S.A.* **76**:5982.

Brockes, J. P., Fields, K. L., and Raff, M. C., 1977, A surface antigenic marker for rat Schwann cells, *Nature (London)* **266**:364.

Brodsky, F. M., Parham, P., Barnstable, C. J., Crumpton, M. J., and Bodmer, W. F., 1979, Monoclonal antibodies for analysis of the HLA system, *Immunol. Rev.* **47**:3.

Burden, S., 1981, Monoclonal antibodies to the frog nerve–muscle synapse, in: *Monoclonal Antibodies to Neural Antigens* (R. McKay, M. C. Raff, and L. F. Reichardt, eds.), p. 247, Cold Spring Harbor Press, Cold Spring Harbor.

Cajal, S. R., 1972, *The Structure of the Retina* (trans. S. A. Thorpe and M. Glickstein), C. C. Thomas, Springfield, Ill.

Carlson, S. S., and Kelly, R. B., 1980, An antiserum specific for cholinergic synaptic vesicles from electric organ, *J. Cell Biol.* **87**:98.

Chaffee, J. K., and Schachner, M., 1978, NS-7 (Nervous System Antigen-7): A cell surface antigen of mature brain, kidney, and spermatozoa shared by embryonal tissues and transformed cells, *Dev. Biol.* **62**:185.

Chalazonitis, A., Greene, L. A., and Shain, W., 1975, Excitability and chemosensitivity properties of a somatic cell hybrid between mouse neuroblastoma and sympathetic ganglion cells, *Exp. Cell Res.* **96**:225.

Cohen, A. I., 1970, Further studies on the question of the potency of saccules in outer segments of vertebrate photoreceptors, *Vision Res.* **10**:445.

Cotton, R. G. H., Secher, D. S., and Milstein, C., 1973, Somatic mutation and the origin of antibody diversity. Clonal variability of the Ig produced by MOPC 21 in culture, *Eur. J. Immunol.* **3**:135.

Dewey, M. M., Davis, P. K., Blasie, J. K., and Barr, L., 1969, Localization of rhodopsin antibody in the retina of the frog, *J. Mol. Biol.* **39**:395.

Eakin, R. M., and Westfall, J. H., 1959, Fine structure of the retina in the reptilian third eye, *J. Biophys. Biochem. Cytol.* **6**:133.

Fazekas de St. Groth, S., and Scheidegger, D., 1980, Production of monoclonal antibodies: Strategy and tactics, *J. Immunol. Methods* **35**:1.

Fekete, D. M., and Barnstable, C. J., 1981, Ultrastructural localisation of rat photoreceptor membrane antigens, submitted for publication.

Galfrè, G., Howe, S. C., Milstein, C., Butcher, G. W., Howard, J. C., 1977, Antibodies to major histocompatibility antigens produced by hybrid cell lines, *Nature (London)* **266**:550.

Hinds, J. W., and Hinds, P. L., 1979, Differentiation of photoreceptors and horizontal cells in the embryonic mouse retina: An electron microscopic, serial section analysis, *J. Comp. Neurol.* **187**:495.

Huttner, W., and Greengard, P., 1979, Multiple phosphorylation sites in protein I and their differential regulation by cyclic AMP and calcium, *Proc. Natl. Acad. Sci. U.S.A.* **76**:5402.

Iversen, L. L., and Kelly, J. S., 1975, Uptake and metabolism of γ-aminobutyric acid by neurones and glial cells, *Biochem. Pharmacol.* **24**:933.

Kearney, J. F., Radbruch, A., Liesegang, B., and Rajewski, K., 1979, A new mouse myeloma cell line that has lost immunoglobulin expression but permits the construction of antibody-secreting hybrid cell lines, *J. Immunol.* **123**:1548.

Kidokoro, Y., Heinemann, S., Schubert, D., Brandt, B. L., and Klier, F. G., 1975, Synapse formation and neurotrophic effects on muscle cell lines, *Cold Spring Harbor Symp. Quant. Biol.* **40**:373.

Köhler, G., and Milstein, C., 1975, Continuous cultures of fused cells secreting antibody of predefined specificity, *Nature (London)* **256**:495.

Kuffler, S. W., Nicholls, J. G., and Orkand, R. K., 1966, Physiological properties of glial cells in the central nervous system of amphibia, *J. Neurophysiol.* **29**:766.

LaVail, M. M., 1976, Survival of some photoreceptor cells in albino rats following long term exposure to continuous light, *Invest. Ophthalmol.* **15**:64.

Letarte-Muirhead, M., Barclay, A. N., and Williams, A. F., 1975, Purification of the Thy-1 molecule, a major cell-surface glycoprotein of rat thymocytes, *Biochem. J.* **151**:685.

Lisak, R. P., Falk, G. A., Heinze, R. G., Kies, M. W., Alvord, E. C., 1970, Dissociation of antibody production from disease suppression in the inhibition of allergic encephalomyelites by myelin basic protein, *J. Immunol.* **104**:1435.

Mendell, J. R., and Whittaker, J. N., 1978, Immunochemical localisation studies of myelin basic protein, *J. Cell Biol.* **76**:502.

Miller, R. E., and Dowling, J. E., 1970, Intracellular responses of the Müller (glial) cells of mudpuppy retina: Their relation to b-wave of the electroretinogram, *J. Neurophysiol.* **33**:323.

Minna, J., Glazer, D., and Nirenberg, M., 1972, Genetic dissection of neural properties using somatic cell hybrids, *Nature (London) New Biol.* **235**:225.

Morris, R. J., and Williams, A. F., 1975, Antigens on mouse and rat lymphocytes recognised by rabbit antiserum against rat brain: The quantitative analysis of a xenogeneic antiserum, *Eur. J. Immunol.* **5**:274.

Moscona, A. A., and Piddington, R., 1966, Stimulation by hydrocortisone of premature changes in the developmental pattern of glutamine synthetase in embryonic retina, *Biochem. Biophys. Acta* **121**:409.

Nilsson, S. E. G., 1964, Receptor cell outer segment development and ultrastructure of the disk membranes in the retina of the tadpole (*Rana pipiens*), *J. Ultrastruct. Res.* **11**:581.

Papermaster, D. S., Schneider, B. G., Zorn, M. A., and Kraekenbull, J. P., 1978, Immunocytochemical localization of a large intrinsic membrane protein to the incisures and margins of frog rod outer segment disks, *J. Cell Biol.* **78**:415.

Parham, P., Barnstable, C. J., and Bodmer, W. F., 1979, Use of a monoclonal antibody (W6/32) in structural studies of HLA-A,B,C antigens, *J. Immunol.* **132**:342.

Peters, A., Palay, S. L., and Webster, H. de F., 1976, *Fine Structure of the* Nervous System, Saunders, Philadelphia.

Raff, M. C., Fields, K. L., Hakomori, S., Mirsky, R., Pruss, R. M., and Winter, J., 1979, Cell-typed-specific markers for distinguishing and studying neurons and the major classes of glial cells in culture, *Brain Res.* **174**:283.

Rutishauser, U., Thiery, J. P., Brackenbury, R., and Edelman, G. M., 1978, Adhesion among neural cells of the chick embryo. III. Relationship of the surface molecule CAM to cell adhesion and development of histaotynic patterns, *J. Cell Biol.* **79**:371.

Sarthy, P. V., and Lam, D. M. K., 1979, Isolated cells from a mammalian retina, *Brain Res.* **176**:208.

Schachner, M., 1974, NS-1 (Nervous System Antigen-1), a glial-cell specific antigenic component of the surface membrane, *Proc. Natl. Acad. Sci. U.S.A.* **71**:1795.

Schechter, I., 1974, Use of antibodies for the isolation of biologically pure messenger ribonucleic acid from fully functional eukaryotic cells, *Biochemistry* **13**:1875.

Schubert, D., Heinemann, S., Carlisle, W., Tarikas, H., Patrick, J., Steinbach, J. H., Culp, W., and Brandt, B. L., 1974, Clonal cell lines from the rat central nervous system, *Nature (London)* **249**:224.

Segal, G. P., and Klinman, N. R., 1976, Defining the heterogeneity of anti-tumor antibody responses, *J. Immunol.* **116**:1539.

Shapiro, D. J., Taylor, J. M., McKnight, G. S., Palacios, R., Gonzalez, C., Kiely, M. L., and Schimke, R. T., 1974, Isolation of hen oviduct ovalbumin and rat liver albumin polysomes by indirect immunoprecipitation, *J. Biol. Chem.* **249**:3665.

Snell, G. D., and Cherry, M., 1972, Loci determining cell surface alloantigens, in *RNA Viruses and Host Genome in Oncogenesis* (P. Emmelot, and P. Bentvelzen, eds.), North-Holland, Amsterdam. pp. 221–228.

Sperry, R. W., 1950, Neuronal specificity, in: *Genetic Neurology* (P. Weiss, ed.), University of Chicago Press, Chicago.

Stallcup, W. B., and Cohn, M., 1976, Correlation of surface antigens and cell type in cloned cell lines from the rat central nervous system, *Exp. Cell Res.* **98**:285.

Sternberger, L. A., 1979, Immunochemistry, 2nd ed., Wiley, New York.

Trisler, G. D., Donlon, M. A., Shain, W. G., and Coon, H. G., 1979, Recognition of antigenic differences among neurons using antiserums to clonal neural retina hybrid cells *Fed. Proc.* **38**:2368.

Uga, S., and Smelser, G. K., 1973a, Electron microscopic study of the development of retinal Müllerian cells, *Invest. Ophthalmol.* **12**:295.

Uga, S., and Smelser, G. K., 1973b, Comparative study of the fine structure of retinal Müller cells in various vertebrates, *Invest. Ophthalmol.* **12**:636.

van de Kamer, J. C., 1965, Histological structure and cytology of the pineal complex in fishes, amphibians and reptiles, *Progr. Brain Res.* **10**:30.

Wacker, W. B., Donoso, L. A., Kalsow, C. M., Yankeelov, J. A., and Organisciak, D. T., 1977, Experimental allergic uveitis. Isolation characterisation and localisation of a soluble uveitopathogenic antigen from bovine retina, *J. Immunol.* **119**:1949.

Williams, A. F., 1977, Differentiation antigens of the lymphocyte cell surface, in: *Contemp. Top. Mol. Immunol.* **6**:93.

Williams, A. F., Galfrè, G., and Milstein, C., 1977, Analysis of cell surfaces by xenogeneic myeloma-hybrid antibodies: Differentiation antigens of rat lymphocytes, *Cell* **12**:663.

Young, R. W., 1968, Passage of newly formed protein through the connecting cilium of retinal rods in the frog, *J. Ultrastruct. Res.* **23**:462.

Yuan, D., Vitetta, E. S., and Schachner, M., 1977, Partial characterization of nervous system-specific cell surface antigen(s) NS-2, *J. Immunol.* **118**:551.

Zimmerman, B. L., and Tso, M. O. M., 1975, Morphologic evidence of photoreceptor differentiation of pinealocytes in the neonatal rat, *J. Cell Biol.* **66**:60.

Zipser, B., and McKay, R., 1981, Monoclonal antibodies distinguish identifiable neurones in the leech, *Nature (London)* **289**:549.

8

Immunological Analysis of Cellular Heterogeneity in the Cerebellum

MELITTA SCHACHNER

1. INTRODUCTION

The complexity of connectivity in the nervous system arises from myriads of associations between different cell types. To investigate the organization of such intricate interconnections the developmental neurobiologist chooses to dissect individual steps in cell–cell interactions during ontogenesis. The assembly of an elaborate system can then be followed from the simple stages through more complex forms to its final state. Underlying these events are several types of cell behavior such as proliferation, growth, and migration; recognition of cellular, extracellular, or subcellular partner components; and often cell death.

The cerebellar cortex provides a favorable scenario in which the formation of individual building blocks can be pursued over time and space. Is is hoped that it might serve as a paradigm in understanding the ontogenesis of other more complex systems which do not have the simple geometry of cell arrangements repeated throughout the cortex and which do not display a similarly protracted developmental time schedule (Eccles *et al.*, 1967; Llinás, 1969; Palay and Chan-Palay, 1974).

MELITTA SCHACHNER · Department of Neurobiology, University of Heidelberg, Heidelberg, Federal Republic of Germany.

The special advantages of the cerebellar cortex in the study of cell–cell interactions are severalfold. It contains relatively few cell types, arranged in three cortical layers—named in order from the outer surface of the folium: the molecular layer, the Purkinje cell layer, and the granular layer which lies adjacent to a stretch of white matter filling the innermost part of a cerebellar folium (Fig. 1). These cytoarchitectonic features are remarkably similar in all vertebrate species (Nieuwenhuys, 1964). The

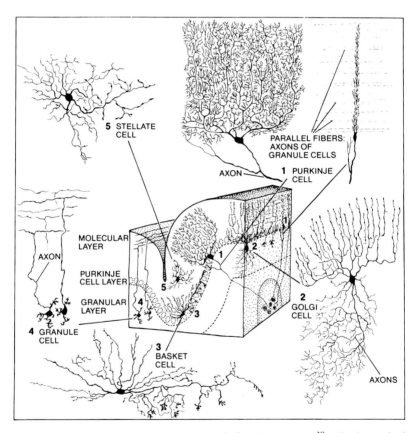

Figure 1. Cerebellar neurons. The human cerebellum has over 10^{10} cells, but only five neuronal types, whose cell bodies are confined to distinct layers; they are shown in drawings made from Golgi-stained preparations. The Purkinje cell (1), whose axons constitute the only output from the cerebellum, has its processes aligned in one plane. The axons of granule cells (4) traverse and make connections with the Purkinje cell process in the molecular layer. The Golgi cell (2), the basket cell (3), and the stellate cell (5) have characteristic positions, shapes, branching patterns, and synaptic connections. (1 and 2) After Ramón y Cajal, 1955; (3–5) after Palay and Chan-Palay, 1974. (From Kuffler and Nicholls, 1976.)

Table I. *Approximate Numerical Relationships between Neuronal Cell Types in Adult Mouse Cerebellum*

Cell type	Relative number
Granule cells	100
Basket and stellate cells	10
Purkinje cells	1
Golgi type II cells	0.1

connectivity and functions of the five neuronal cell types, the Purkinje, stellate, basket, Golgi type II, and granule cells are known in considerable detail. The Purkinje cell is the principal neuron and the sole efferent pathway of the cerebellum. The interneurons or local circuit neurons, so called because all their synaptic partners lie within the cortex itself, are the stellate, basket, Golgi type II, and granule cells. In mammals some major events in neuron formation and migration as well as overt synaptogenesis take place postnatally so they become easily amenable to experimental analysis.

Cerebellar ontogenesis follows a rather invariant time schedule. Large neurons, the Purkinje and Golgi type II neurons, are generated first, mainly between embryonic days 11 and 13 in the mouse (Miale and Sidman, 1961), followed by the genesis of stellate, basket, and granule cells, which lasts from postnatal day 4 to approximately day 14. These two cell groups originate from distinct germinal zones. A zone in the roof of the fourth ventricle gives rise to Purkinje and Golgi type II cells as well as glial cells, some of which are to become a particular class of astrocytes, the Bergmann glial cells, also known as Golgi epithelial cells. These cells migrate outward from the ventricular zone of the fourth ventricle to form the mantle layer of the cerebellar plate. Another germinal zone, the external granular layer, forms beneath the external surface of the cerebellar anlage to give rise to stellate, basket, and the large number of granule cells, which eventually make up about 90% of all cerebellar neurons (Table I). Some glia may also derive from this germinal zone.

The external granular layer constitutes a secondary matrix zone which receives its cell population from the rostral part of the rhombic lip, a germinal zone in the alar plate forming the wall of the fourth ventricle (Schaper, 1894a,b; Ramón y Cajal, 1909–1911; Raaf and Kernohan, 1944). In all vertebrates the external granular layer increases in thickness as a result of proliferation of the germinal external granule cells (Uzman, 1960; Fujita, 1967; Mareš et al., 1970). During the initial increase in thickness all granule cells engage in DNA synthesis, as was shown by Fujita and colleagues by cumulative labeling with [³H]thymidine (Fujita et al., 1966). After this initial period of cell proliferation, the inner portion of cells in the external granular layer lying between the actively proliferating external granule cells and the Purkinje cells withdraws from the cell cycle. These postmitotic granule cells extend two bipolar axonal processes oriented parallel to the surface of the cerebellar cortex in the direction of the folia. The granule cell body attaches to the radial process of a Bergmann glial cell and migrates inward from the external surface following its leading process in a straight radial pathway. In this passage the Bergmann glia act as contact guideposts through a territory apparently blocked by obstacles in the form of earlier generated cells and cellular processes (Mugnaini and Forströnen, 1967; Rakic, 1971). Migration of granule cells is completed by detachment from the Bergmann glia and assumption of the final position in the internal granular layer. The granule cells which are generated and migrate first are situated deepest in the cerebellar cortex. Granule cells which become postmitotic in progressively superficial strata of the external granular layer form their axonal processes in these more superficial parts apposing the parallel fibers of previously elaborated granule cell axons. These later-generated granule cells assume correspondingly more superficial positions in the internal granular layer, resulting in an "inside out" pattern (Rakic, 1972, 1973). Like the granule cells, basket and stellate neurons derive from the external granular layer but migrate only as far as the molecular layer.

As a result of the differential generation in time of the two groups of cerebellar neurons, selective damage and destruction of cell classes can be achieved by radiation (Hicks and D'Amato, 1966; Altman and Anderson, 1972), viruses (Kilham and Margolis, 1966a,b; Herndon et al., 1971a,b), and chemical agents (Hicks, 1954; Herndon, 1968; Nathanson et al., 1969; Shimada and Langman, 1970; Zamenhof et al., 1971; Webster et al., 1973), some of which were shown to interfere with DNA synthesis. When administered at the early postnatal times during active proliferation of external granule cells, the cerebellar cortex develops without granule, stellate, and basket cell neurons. Such experimental manipulation of cortical histogenesis offers special advantages in the study of adaptation in neuronal connectivity to epigenetically induced abnormalities in cellular milieu.

In addition to such exogenous disruptions of cortical development, even greater advantages for investigations of cerebellar ontogenesis derive from the availability of neurological mutations of the mouse, which generally affect cell migration and differentiation but not proliferation and time of origin (Sidman et al., 1965). Four mutations affecting the cerebellum will be described in more detail here, since they will be referred to later in this article.

1.   *reeler* (Falconer, 1951; Mariani et al., 1977; Caviness and Rakic, 1979). Reeler mice are characterized behaviorally by ataxia, fine tremor, and hypotonia. The cerebellum is reduced in size, and folia are practically absent. Purkinje cells display their characteristic, although somewhat stunted, dendritic arbor and are grossly misplaced throughout the vestigial cerebellum. The number of granule cells is reduced. Most granule cells lie in the superficial parts of the abnormal cerebellum, which lacks the laminar structure of cortical layers. Despite the cellular disorder, synaptic associations between misplaced and disoriented neurons appear comparatively normal.

2.   *weaver* (Lane, 1964; Sidman, 1968; Rezai and Yoon, 1972; Rakic and Sidman, 1973; Hirano and Dembitzer, 1973; Sotelo and Changeux, 1974b; Sotelo, 1975a,b; Caviness and Rakic, 1978). Similar to reeler, homozygous weaver mice are hypotonic and ataxic and have fine tremor. The cerebellum is small due to the degeneration of granule cells during the 2nd and 3rd postnatal week. The primary defect in weaver was sought in the Bergmann glia by Rakic and Sidman because morphological abnormalities in these cells were the earliest detectable within the first postnatal days. However, it is also possible that the primary genetic defect is closer to the granule cell as Sotelo and Changeux have proposed. As a result of the abnormal relationship between external granule cells and Bergmann glia, granule cells fail to migrate and die, probably as a consequence of this failure.

3.   *staggerer* (Sidman et al., 1962; Sotelo and Changeux, 1974a; Landis and Sidman, 1974; Sotelo, 1975a; Landis and Reese, 1977; Caviness and Rakic, 1978). Clinically similar to the aforementioned mutants, the staggerer mutant is deficient in Purkinje cell deployment. The Purkinje cells are either absent or have stunted dendrites which are devoid of spines. Granule cells are born and migrate normally but start to degenerate during the second postnatal week. There are no Purkinje cell–parallel fiber synapses. It has therefore been suggested that granule cells degenerate because they depend on the interaction with their postsynaptic partners, the Purkinje cells. Purkinje cells survive, however, more successfully in the absence of granule cell inputs.

4.   *Purkinje cell degeneration* (Mullen et al., 1976; Landis and Mullen, 1978; Caviness and Rakic, 1978). In the mutant Purkinje cell degeneration, cerebellar ontogenesis proceeds normally until the beginning of the 3rd postnatal week, when Purkinje cells start to degenerate. During

the 3rd week, when most of the distal dendritic segments of Purkinje cells are developing, spines do not develop. By the end of the 4th postnatal week virtually all Purkinje cells have been lost. Despite the loss of the only efferent cerebellar pathway, Purkinje cell degeneration is behaviorally less severely affected than the other mutants described above.

In this chapter I wish to focus on the description of cell-type-specific markers recognized and characterized by antibodies as immunological reagents. The expression of these markers will be followed as a function of development from embryonic stages to adulthood. It is anticipated that through the precise definition of cell-type-specific markers it will be possible to isolate cerebellar cell types as homogeneous populations and use these populations to study selected individual steps in cell–cell interactions *in vitro* both in normal and in genetically abnormal situations. It should be possible not only to make use of immunoselective methods *in vitro*, but to employ antibody mediated cytolysis *in situ* to study the effects of a loss of individual cell populations on the interactions between the residual cell types. It is only through a complete account of each individual cell type, and even subsets within a particular cell type, throughout development that the problem of origin and cell lineage relationships will be solved, and a dissection of cellular heterogeneity in the cerebellum will be achieved.

The availability of refined immunological methodology is imperative for the recognition of subtle molecular differences and similarities among neural cell classes. Most neural antigens have so far been defined by xenogeneic antisera for which species differences exist between the animal yielding tissue or cells for immunization and the immunized host animal. To render the resulting antisera specific for nervous tissue and/or neural cell type, antibodies to species-specific antigens which are not of interest have to be removed by extensive absorption with non-neural tissues. Even though operationally specific antisera could thus be obtained, they are most likely still heterogeneous with respect to antigenic specificities, antibody subclasses, and binding affinities.

Monoclonal antibodies, which can be obtained with relative ease by the myeloma-hybrid technique of Köhler and Milstein (1975, 1976), circumvent these various problems of conventional antisera. In cases when complex mixtures of antigens are used for immunization, monoclonal antibodies are able to dissect this heterogeneity and potentially enable the detection of minor antigens and minor cell populations when appropriate assay systems are used. This approach has opened new avenues in the investigation of neural cell types and the characterization of more refined differences among developing and adult cells.

2. GLIAL MARKERS

All classes of glia as well as neurons presumably originate from a common stem cell, the germinal cell (His, 1889), which constitutes the epithilium of the neural tube. It is not known when the program of differential gene expression is initiated in the neuroepithelium and when the differentiative pathways of neurons and glia, and subsets within glia, diverge from each other. The origin of glia is particularly difficult to trace in development since, in contrast to neurons, they continue to proliferate often throughout life (Smart and Leblond, 1961; Privat, 1975). An orderly sequence of growth and differentiation of glia and glial subpopulations has therefore yet to become apparent. The two types of macroglia seem to arise from a common precursor, the glioblast (Schaper, 1897a,b). Whether these are pluripotential glial cells capable of differentiating into both oligodendroglia as well as astroglia, or whether they constitute distinct subsets of glial precursors, is presently undecided.

The problem of origin and differentiation of glial cells has been hampered both by the lack of understanding of glial functions and by the fact that unequivocal criteria for identification of glia at early developmental stages have not been established. In addition to the sometimes problematic ultrastructural description, biochemical markers detectable by specific and sensitive immunological reagents are needed. Furthermore, such reagents are called for when cell types have to be identified in culture, where a cell's characteristic morphology can be grossly altered.

As a major subclass of glial cells, astroglia have been known for more than a century. Their functional role in cell–cell interactions has, however, remained largely obscure. They may provide nutritive and structural support for neurons and may be instrumental in both chemical and physical isolation of neurons and their synapses (for review, see Peters et al., 1976). They have been shown to retain the ability to divide and grow in response to neural damage (Maxwell and Krüger, 1965; Huntington and Terry, 1966; Vaughn et al., 1970). Radial astroglial processes in the developing brain have been proposed to act as guides for migrating neurons in the cerebellar and cerebral cortices (Rakic, 1971; Schmechel and Rakic, 1979). This neuron–glia relationship might be disturbed in the weaver mutant, as has been mentioned in Section 1.

Historically, astroglia have been divided into two subclasses. Astrocytes in white-matter regions abound in intermediate-sized filaments and have therefore been designated fibrillary or fibrous astrocytes. Protoplasmic astrocytes with more attenuated processes are typical for gray-matter regions and contain relatively fewer filaments. It is not known at present whether these two types of astrocytes display distinct functional traits. Both are characterized by the expression of glial fibrillary acidic (GFA) protein, which is found in astrocytes but no other neural or nonneural cell type in the CNS (Eng *et al.*, 1971; Bignami *et al.*, 1972). This protein of an apparent molecular mass of 54,000 daltons is the presumed monomeric subunit of 100-Å, intermediate-sized filaments. Its function is presently unknown.

As a second major subclass of macroglia, oligodendrocytes have been distinguished by distinct structural and functional features (for review, see Peters *et al.*, 1976). The immature form, the oligodendroglioblast, so called because of its ability to proliferate, undergoes morphologically distinct transitions to mature forms which generally cease to divide and are capable of myelination. Myelination is the last of these differentiative steps and possibly the most complex. The cellular mechanisms of proliferation and differentiation of oligodendroglia, particularly their communication with nerve axons, have remained largely obscure.

2.1. Astroglial Antigens

Beside the now classical marker for astrocytes in the postnatal CNS, GFA protein, a novel marker for astroglia in the embryonic and adult neuroectoderm, has emerged in the form of vimentin, formerly found to be expressed predominantly in cells of mesenchymal origin (Franke *et al.*, 1978). Furthermore, two other intracellular antigens detected by monoclonal antibodies will be described. They are differentially distributed among astroglial subclasses in cerebellum and other parts of the CNS. These have been called M1 and C1 antigens. A cell surface antigen detected by a xenogeneic antiserum to bovine corpus callosum and present on both astroglia and oligodendroglia has been described previously (Schachner *et al.*, 1977; Campbell *et al.*, 1977).

2.1.1. Vimentin (Schnitzer et al., 1981) (see Tables II–V). Vimentin is the protein subunit of a type of intermediate-sized filament characterized originally in mesenchymal tissues of vertebrates. The antiserum was prepared in guinea pigs to murine vimentin and purified by affinity chromatography to yield a specific immunoglobulin fraction. The expression of vimentin in the nervous system, particularly the cerebellum, was studied in histological sections and in monolayer cultures. To identify cell types and correlate staining patterns, vimentin is immunolabeled with the fluorescin fluorochrome, while another independent marker previously established to be cell type specific is labeled with rhodamine.

One and the same part of a histological section or culture can then be viewed simultaneously by simply changing filters of the fluorescence microscope. In addition, the phase contrast image can be used for reference.

In such double immunolabeling experiments, GFA protein serves as a marker for the more mature astrocytes in the mouse cerebellum which become detectable approximately at the end of the 1st postnatal week (Lagenaur et al., 1980). Fetal cerebellar astrocytes do not express GFA protein at levels detectable by indirect immunofluorescence methods. To recognize oligodendroglia, galactocerebroside and NS-1 antisera were used (Schachner and Willinger, 1979a,b; Raff et al., 1979a).

Antibodies to fibronectin served to mark fibroblasts and fibroblastlike cells (Schachner and Willinger, 1979a; Schachner et al., 1978b). Recently another cell surface component of mesodermally derived cells, laminin (Timpl et al., 1979), has been found to be expressed on fibronectin-positive cells (M. Schachner, unpublished results). It is not known at present if fibroblastlike cells with their characteristic epithelioid morphology in monolayer cultures are the typical fibroblasts of connective tissue present in meninges and choroid plexus, or if some of these cells are of endothelial or possibly ependymal origin, since individual markers for each of these cell types alone have not yet been found. In immunoelectronmicroscopic studies of intact tissue, both endothelial and ependymal cells are stained by antiserum to fibronection at the lumen-facing side (Schachner et al., 1978b).

Tetanus toxin and NS-4 antiserum were used to stain neurons *in situ* and *in vitro*, where at low cell densities and after culture periods of less than 4–6 weeks predominantly neurons are labeled (Dimpfel et al., 1977; Mirsky et al., 1978; Schachner et al., 1975; Rohrer and Schachner, 1980; Schnitzer and Schachner, 1981a,b).

In histological sections of adult mouse cerebellum vimentin is expressed in astrocytes and ependymal cells, but not in neurons or oligodendrocytes. Vimentin appears also be be detectable in the mesodermally derived parts of choroid plexus and meninges. Whether vimentin is also expressed in choroid epithelial or leptomeningeal cells will have to be investigated by immunoelectron microscopy. Interestingly, vimentin is not recognizable in cerebellar endothelial cells, although it has been detected in cultured endothelial cells of human origin (Franke et al., 1979). Larger blood vessels are, however, amply stained by vimentin antiserum. (See Fig. 2 for illustrations.)

Specific labeling of all GFA-protein-positive astrocytes, but not of neurons or oligodendroglia, is confirmed in primary cultures of early postnatal mouse cerebellum (Fig. 3). Fibronectin-positive fibroblasts or

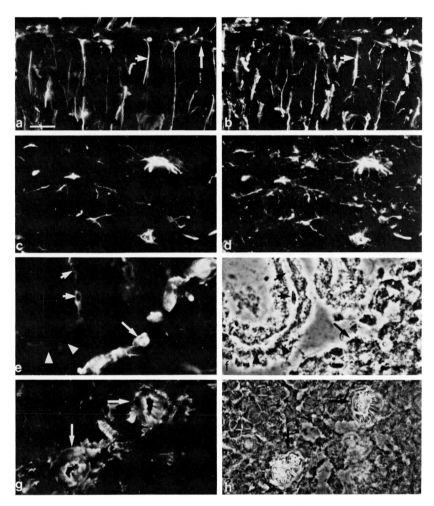

Figure 2. Immunofluorescence microscopy on frozen sagittal sections of adult C57BL/6J mouse brain. (a, b) Double immunolabeling of the cerebellar molecular layer for vimentin (a) (fluorescein) and GFA protein (b) (rhodamine). (a) and (b) represent identical visual fields. Meninges are marked by large arrows, radially oriented fibers by small arrows. (c, d) Double immunolabeling of the cerebellar white matter for vimentin (c) and GFA protein (d). As in (a) and (b), vimentin seems to be restricted more to the sturdier cellular processes and is hardly detected in the finer GFA-protein-positive extensions. (e) Immunolabeling of ependyma and choroid plexus of the fourth ventricle for vimentin. Positive reaction is seen in ependymal cells (large arrows) and in some inner portions of the plexus (small arrows). Choroid epithelial cells are vimentin negative (arrowheads). (f) Phase contrast micrograph of fluorescent picture (e). (g) Immunolabeling of large blood vessels (arrows) for vimentin. (h) Phase contrast micrograph of fluorescent picture (g). Bar denotes 20μm. (From Schnitzer et al., 1981.)

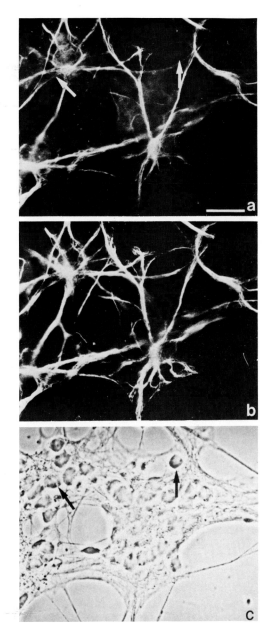

Figure 3. Double immunolabeling of vimentin (a) (fluorescein) and GFA protein (b) (rhodamine) in 3-day cultures of cells from 7-day C57BL/6J mouse cerebellum. Vimentin-positive cells (a) are also labeled by antibodies to GFA protein (b); cells with small cell bodies (arrows), probably granule cell neurons, are not stained. (c) Phase contrast micrograph. Bar denotes 20 μm. (From Schnitzer et al., 1981.)

fibroblastlike cells also express vimentin (Figs. 4 and 5). These two cell populations are not only vimentin positive in cultures of early postnatal cerebellum, but also at embryonic ages. Since the cerebellar anlage at embryonic day 13, when the first neurons are born, contains very few cells, other brain parts were taken for monolayer cultures. In cultures

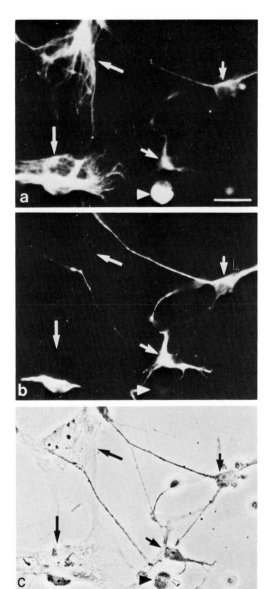

Figure 4. Double immunolabeling of vimentin (a) (fluorescein) and GFA protein (b) (rhodamine) in 3-day cultures of cells from 7-day C57BL/6J mouse cerebellum. Vimentin-positive cells (a) include GFA-protein-positive astrocytes (b) (small arrows), GFA-protein-negative cells with fibroblastlike morphology (large arrows), and an unidentified GFA-protein-negative cell type with round cell soma (arrowhead), possibly an ependymal cell. (c) Phase contrast micrograph. Bar denotes 20 μm. (From Schnitzer et al., 1981.)

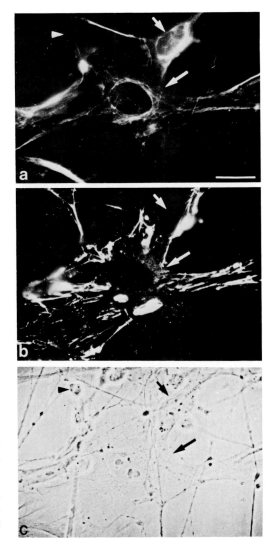

Figure 5. Double immunolabeling of vimentin (a) (fluorescein) and fibronectin (b) (rhodamine) in 3-day cultures of cells from 6-day C57BL/6J mouse cerebellum. A vimentin-positive cell with fibroblastlike morphology (a) (large arrow) is also positive for fibronectin (b). Another vimentin-positive cell (a) (small arrow) located on top of the fibroblastlike cell is not stained by fibronectin antibodies (b). Cells with small cell bodies (a) (arrowheads), probably granule cell neurons, are not stained with either antibody. (c) Phase contrast micrograph. Bar denotes 20 μm. (From Schnitzer et al., 1981.)

of embryonic day 11 telencephalon (embryonic day 0 is counted as the day a vaginal plug is found), vimentin is never expressed in cells which carry receptors for tetanus toxin or express neurofilament antigen, the subunit protein of intermediate-sized filaments in neurons. In addition to fibronectin, NS-4 antigen, tetanus toxin receptors, and neurofilament are the only markers for neuroectodermal cells which at present are expressed at this early developmental stage (Schachner et al., 1979b; Schnitzer and Schachner, 1981c). A direct demonstration of vimentin

Table II. Expression of Glial Antigens in Adult and Embryonic Mouse Cerebellum

Antigen	Adult	Embryonic
C1	+	+
M1	+	−
Vimentin	+	+
GFA protein	+	−

expression in astroglia was not feasible at embryonic ages, since conventional astrocytic markers are not yet expressed. With a novel marker for embryonic astroglia, the C1 antigen, coincident expression of radial glial fibers with vimentin can be demonstrated in histological sections.

2.1.2. *C1 Antigen* (Sommer et al., 1981; Sommer and Schachner, 1981c) (see Tables II–V). A monoclonal antibody designated anti-C1 was produced by a hybridoma clone from a fusion of NS1 myeloma with spleen cells of BALB/c mice injected with homogenate of white matter from bovine corpus callosum. This source of antigen was chosen because conventionally prepared polyclonal antibodies reacted with cell surfaces of astrocytes as well as oligodendrocytes, and it was hoped that it would be possible to dissect this apparent heterogeneity by monoclonal antibodies.

In the adult mouse cerebellum, C1 antigen is detectable in the processes of Bergmann glial cells, but not in astrocytes of the granular layer or white matter (Fig. 6). Another type of astrocyte with radially oriented processes, the Müller cell in the retina, is also positive for C1, whereas GFA-protein-positive astrocytes in the ganglion cell layer do not express C1. Other regions of the CNS have yet to be studied systematically for C1 expression, but so far most astrocytes, including those with radial glial processes in the area dentata of the hippocampus, have all been

Table III. Cellular Localization of Glial Antigens in Adult Mouse Neuroectoderm

Antigen	Cellular localization
C1	Radial astroglia in cerebellum and retina; ependyma
M1	All astrocytes in white-matter areas; astrocytes in area dentata of the hippocampus and their radial processes; astrocytes in ganglion cell layer of the retina
Vimentin	All astrocytes; ependyma
GFA protein	All astrocytes

Table IV. Localization of Glial Antigens in Developing Mouse Neuroectoderm

Antigen	Embryonic CNS	Early postnatal cerebellum
C1	Radial fibers	Bergmann glia; astrocytes in white matter and developing internal granular layer
M1	Negative	Bergmann glia; astrocytes in white matter and developing internal granular layer
Vimentin	Radial fibers; ventricular cells	Astroglia; ependyma
GFA protein	Negative (in cerebellum)	Astroglia

found negative for C1. Similar to vimentin, C1 is expressed in most if not all ependymal cells, in fibroblasts or fibroblastlike cells in culture, and in larger blood vessels, but not in capillaries. It seems to be localized intracellularly.

In the developing, early postnatal cerebellum, C1 is not confined to Bergmann glia and ependymal cells, but is additionally present in astrocytes of presumptive white matter and Purkinje cell layer. Still earlier in development, C1 is expressed already at embryonic day 11, the earliest stage tested so far. At this stage C1 is expressed in radial glial fibers in telencephalon, pons, and anlage of pituitary and retina, thus resembling vimentin. Unlike vimentin, however, C1 is not expressed in ventricular cells at this age.

This cellular pattern of C1 expression is suggestive of particular

Table V. Expression of Glial Antigens in Neurological Mouse Mutants Purkinje cell degeneration, reeler, staggerer, and weaver[a]

Antigen	Cerebellum	Retina
C1	Bergmann glia negative (abnormal); ependyma positive (normal)	Müller cells positive (normal)
M1	Early postnatal pattern (abnormal)	Astrocytes in ganglion cell layer positive (normal)
Vimentin	All astrocytes and ependyma positive (normal)	All astrocytes positive (normal)
GFA protein	All astrocytes positive (normal)	All astrocytes positive (normal)

[a] Ages of mice: reeler and staggerer, approximately 3 weeks; Purkinje cell degeneration, approximately 3 months; weaver, approximately 5 months.

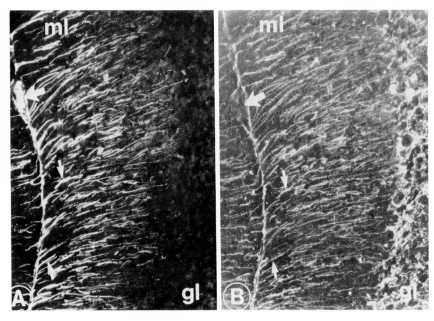

Figure 6. Immunohistological staining of C1 antigen and GFA protein in the cerebellar cortex of an adult C57BL/6J mouse. (A) C1 antigen is detected in radial Bergmann glial fibers in the molecular layer (ml). The meninges-proximal portions of these fibers are more heavily stained with C1 antibodies (A) (see small arrows) than with GFA protein antiserum (B), which labels Bergmann fibers more uniformly throughout the molecular layer. The granular layer (gl) is negative for C1 antigen (A), but positive for GFA protein (B). A larger blood vessel in the meninges is stained by C1 antibodies (A) (see large arrow), but not with GFA protein antiserum (B). × 220, reproduced at 75%. (From Sommer *et al.*, 1981.)

structural and functional relationships between ependyma, embryonic radial glial fibers, and a certain population of astrocytes comprising Bergmann glia and Müller cells with their radially oriented cellular processes, but not the radial astroglia in the hippocampus. Radial glia in the cerebellum and retina appear to be direct descendants of the primitive embryonic radial glia, the processes of which span the neural tube from ventricular lumen to surface. While Müller cells remain attached to the outer and inner surfaces of the neuroectoderm at adult stages, Bergmann glia lose their connection to the inner surface in many vertebrates and retain solely their apposition to the pial surface. The radial fibers of astrocytes in the area dentata of the hippocampus arise after the disappearance of primitive glial processes (A. Privat, personal communication) by the subsequent elaboration of secondary processes, an event which has been described for the formation of protoplasmic astrocytes in the occipital lobe of the monkey (Schmechel and Rakic, 1979). It seems plausible, therefore, to speculate that the descendants of primitive radial glia retain features in common with their precursors and that C1 antigen might be an indicator of such a relationship.

Expression of C1 in ependymal cells would indicate that these share common properties with astrocytes, as suggested by several authors using ultrastructural criteria (for reviews, see Peters *et al.*, 1976; Oksche, 1980). The fact that ependymal cells in higher vertebrates retain some properties of primitive glia is evidenced by the existence of tanycytes of the third ventricle. These cells span the neuroectoderm at adult stages and are therefore presumed to unite glial and ependymal properties in one cell type (Oksche, 1980). Indeed, in the frog *Rana pipiens* ependymal cells have been found to span the cerebellar cortex even at adult stages, thus substituting for the classical Bergmann glia, which are absent in these animals (Korte and Rosenbluth, 1980). In adult lower vertebrates the so-called ependymal glial cells are able to form intercellular channels in the neighborhood of a lesion (Egar and Singer, 1972; Nordlander and Singer, 1978). These channels are reminiscent of those described for ependymal cells at embryonic stages of lower vertebrates, as well as for the primitive glia of higher vertebrates (Silver and Robb, 1979; Silver and Sidman, 1980), and are presumed to function as contact guideposts for the outgrowing axonal processes. In the mouse, these channels seem to originate as spaces between radially oriented primitive glia. The capacity to reform these channels in ependymal cells during spinal cord regeneration appears to be suppressed or lost in mammals. It seems, however, that mature ependyma in adult higher vertebrates express at least one property suggestive of a more primitive potential—the expression of C1 antigen and also vimentin.

Because of the early expression of C1 in morphogentically active cells, such as the primitive radial glia and Bergmann glia, it seemed pertinent to investigate C1 expression in the weaver mutant, which shows abnormal interaction between Bergmann glia and granule cells during the migratory phase. It was indeed found by immunohistological methods that in the adult weaver cerebellum C1 is not detectable in Bergmann glia, but readily detected in ependymal cells of the fourth ventricle, as it is in the wild type. This abnormality in C1 expression is not confined, however, to the weaver mutant, but is also observed in three other cerebellar mutants tested so far. These are staggerer, reeler, and Purkinje cell degeneration, which display a broad spectrum of cerebellar abnormalities differing not only from the weaver mutation, but also from each other. In these mutants C1 is still detectable in the cerebellum and in Bergmann glial processes at postnatal day 7, but disappears during the 2nd postnatal week in reeler, staggerer and weaver. Regions of the cerebellum which mature earlier under normal conditions are the first ones to lose C1 in these three mutants. Reeler, in which morphological abnormalities are manifest at fetal ages, is the first mutant to lose C1. It is followed by weaver and then staggerer. The order of disappearance of C1 antigen is parallel to the onset of the morphologically recognizable abnormality. In Purkinje cell degeneration, the disappearance of C1 is delayed until the 4th postnatal week, possibly reflecting a later onset in the manifestation of the abnormal phenotype. Moreover, expression of vimentin is not detectably affected in any of the GFA-protein-positive populations of cerebellar astrocytes.

It is difficult to reconcile these observations with a unifying hypothesis. The simplest explanation would be to link a more general type of cellular abnormality or trauma (Lagenaur et al., 1980) to the suppression of C1 expression, which occurs normally up to a certain age but then declines. It is noteworthy that in three mutants, the disappearance of C1 expression coincides with the time in the normal cerebellum when Bergmann glia cease to proliferate and the migratory activity of granule cells is at its peak (Das, 1974). The abnormality of cerebellar development in reeler seems to occur well before this time, during the second trimester of fetal life. In weaver, ultrastructural abnormalities in Bergmann glia become evident during the 1st postnatal week. In staggerer, migration of granule cells is not affected, but cell death occurs soon afterward. Purkinje cell degeneration loses C1 expression later than the aforementioned mutants, and at a time when almost all Purkinje cells have degenerated. Interestingly, Müller cells normally express C1 in this mutant at times when loss of retinal photoreceptor cells is underway (Mullen and La Vail, 1975). In the future it will be important to investigate the parameters involved in the regulation of C1 synthesis and degradation under pathological conditions not only in vivo, but also in vitro.

2.1.3. *M1 Antigen* (Lagenaur et al., 1980) (see Tables II–V). This antigen is recognized by a monoclonal antibody produced by a hybridoma that arose from the fusion of NS1 myeloma and splenocytes derived from a Sprague–Dawley rat immunized with a crude membrane fraction of early postnatal C57BL/6J mouse cerebella.

By indirect immunohistology in adult mouse cerebellum, only astrocytes in white matter can be shown to contain M1. Astrocytes in granular, Purkinje cell and molecular layers are not positive for M1. During development, M1 is first detectable at approximately postnatal day 7 in white matter astrocytes. At postnatal day 10, M1 is additionally present in Bergmann glial fibers and in astrocytes of the developing internal granular layer (Fig. 7). M1 expression in these latter astrocytes is transient and disappears by the 4th postnatal week, when the general maturation of the mouse cerebellum has reached completion. Like C1, M1 seems to be expressed intracellularly.

Both M1 and GFA protein serve as markers for the more mature, differentiated astrocytes at postnatal ages, whereas vimentin and C1 are characteristically expressed at the early developmental stages of primitive astroblasts.

The exact time at which vimentin and C1 antigen become expressed remains to be determined. It is also unclear if all astroblasts express vimentin and C1, and if these two antigens mark the appearance of a distinct lineage of astrocytic macroglia at the point of divergence from neuroblasts and oligodendroblasts. It is conceivable that C1 is expressed even in the common precursor or stem cells to all neural cell types, and

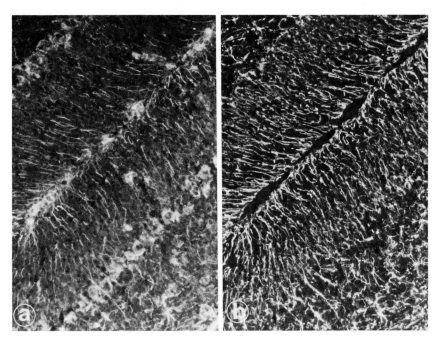

Figure 7. Immunofluorescent staining of M1 antigen and GFA protein in cerebellar cortex of 10-day C57BL/6J mice. At postnatal day 10, M1 antigen is prominent in Purkinje cell bodies (large arrow) and astrocytes of white matter, and granular and molecular layers (a). Some Bergmann fibers and astroglia in the granular layer that are detectable by anti-GFA protein antiserum appear M1 antigen negative. Some staining of blood vessels in the meninges (small arrows) is also seen. (a) M1 antigen (fluorescein); (b) GFA protein (rhodamine). × 220, reproduced at 75%. (From Lagenaur et al., 1980.)

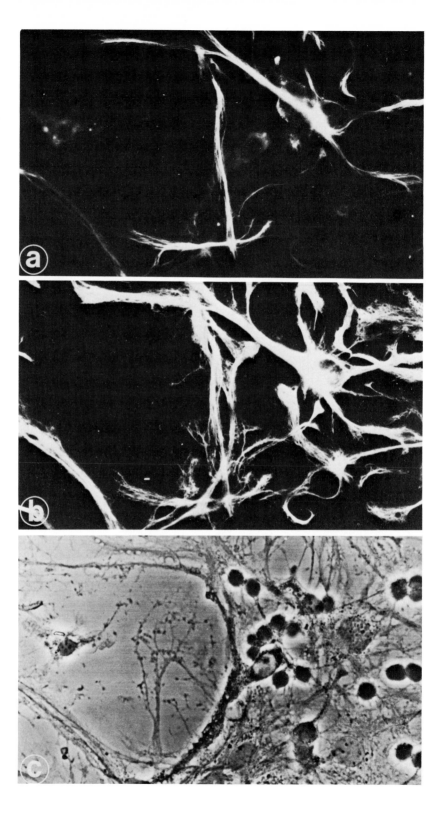

later becomes restricted to a particular subclass as has been suggested for vimentin (Tapscott *et al.*, 1980). The phenomenon of vimentin-positive ventricular cells will have to be investigated using electron-microscopic methods and ultrastructural features as guidelines.

In contrast to the early markers vimentin and C1, M1 and GFA protein appear in the late stages of astrocyte differentiation. The regulation of M1 expression in the cerebellum differs in several respects, however, from that of GFA protein. Expression of GFA protein is first detectable at postnatal day 2 in the peduncular parts of the cerebellum, and precedes the appearance of M1, which first becomes detectable on day 7 in these areas. the transient expression of M1 in astrocytes of granular and molecular layers does not seem to occur in all GFA-protein-positive astrocytes. This phenomenon is also reflected in monolayer cultures of early postnatal mouse cerebellum, where M1 is apparent in a subpopulation of GFA-protein-positive astrocytes (Fig. 8). It is unlikely that M1-positive astrocytes are lost through cell death *in situ*, since M1 can be seen to disappear gradually in astrocytes, while GFA protein continues to be expressed without apparent decrement in the identical cell population. It seems, therefore, that even at relatively late stages of differentiation, expression of an astrocyte marker is under developmental regulation. It remains to be seen which factors influence expression of M1 antigen at these stages *in situ* and *in vitro*.

Four cerebellar mutants—reeler, staggerer, weaver, and Purkinje cell degeneration—were studied to gain insight into the regulation of M1 expression. In all four mutants, M1 was observed to persist into adulthood in Bergmann glia and other astrocytes which normally do not express it. It therefore seems as if these mutants are not capable of repressing M1 in Bergmann glia as part of their developmental program, but continue to remain in an immature state. It is quite unlikely that this apparent blockage in maturation of some astrocytes represents a direct effect of mutant genes on particular astrocytes. It might, however, indicate a more general response to a pathological situation in the form of an abnormal cellular environment (Lagenaur *et al.*, 1981), as has been hypothesized for C1 antigen. Reminiscent of C1 is also the observation that M1 is expressed normally in adult retina, where it is confined to astrocytes in the ganglion cell layer but absent from Müller cells. These express C1 equally well in the mutant and wild type.

←――

Figure 8. Immunoflorescent staining of M1 antigen and GFA protein in monolayer cultures of cerebellar cells from 6-day C57BL/6J mice. Cells were maintained for 3 days in culture, fixed with paraformaldehyde and acetone, and double labeled with anti-M1 and anti-GFA protein antibodies. Some, but not all, cells and cellular processes that are GFA protein positive are also M1 antigen positive. (a) M1 antigen (fluorescein); (b) GFA protein (rhodamine). (c) Phase contrast photomicrograph. × 560. (From Lagenaur *et al.*, 1980.)

It seems pertinent now to ask if C1 and M1 antigens are expressed in a mutually exclusive fashion in astroglia of the adult cerebellum and nervous system. Although C1 and M1 have not been observed in one and the same cell, they are not strictly complementary to each other, since astrocytes have been found which express neither of the two antigen, e.g., astrocytes in the cerebellar granular layer. It is furthermore worth pointing out that the two antigens do not fit the categories of fibrillary and protoplasmic astrocytes. For instance, M1 is expressed not only in the fibrillary astrocytes of cerebellar white matter, but also in protoplasmic astrocytes of the area dentata in the hippocampus and their radial processes. Similarly, C1 is present in only a small fraction of protoplasmic astrocytes, which are, as far as we have been able to study them, the cerebellar Bergmann glia and the retinal Müller cells.

In conclusion, the two intracellular markers C1 and M1 characterize two distinct types of astroglia which do not conform to the conventional classification of protoplasmic and fibrillary astrocytes. The antigens show a divergent differentiative potential, which has been distinguished biochemically for the first time. C1 is characteristic of primitive radial glia and their direct descendants. M1 characterizes astroglia derived from these primitive glia by morphological transformation. Abnormal expression of antigens in the pathological situations of mutation and experimental trauma seems to indicate also distinct functional properties: M1 expression is enhanced in astroglia which normally do not express it, while C1 is suppressed. It seems therefore possible that M1 signifies the "reactive" state of astroglia, during development and at adult stages, while C1 might be characteristic of a more primitive, "morphogenetic" potential in astroglia, which is lost under pathological conditions.

2.2. Oligodendroglial Antigens

2.2.1. O Antigens (O1–O4) (Sommer and Schachner, 1981; Schachner et al., 1981; Berg and Schachner, 1981) (see Tables VI and VII). Four monoclonal antibodies designated O1, O2, O3, and O4 have been obtained which react with the cell surfaces of oligodendroglia. The antibody-secreting hybridoma clones were derived from a fusion of NS1 myeloma with splenocytes from BALB/c mice immunized with white matter of bovine corpus callosum. The antibodies were first recognized by screening hybridoma supernatants on fresh-frozen sections of adult mouse cerebellum by indirect immunofluorescence. Staining of white matter tracts was prominent with all four antibodies, but additional immunolabeling was visible in round or oval membranous material stained with O2, O3, and O4 antibodies (Fig. 9). Radially oriented Berg-

Table VI. *Percentage of O-Antigen-Positive Cells Expressing Cell-Type-Specific Markers*[a]

Cell-type-specific marker	Antigen			
	01	02	03	04
GFA protein	0	0	0	0
Tetanus toxin receptors	0	0	0	0
Fibronectin	0	0	0	0
Galactocerebroside	100 ± 10	90 ± 8	65 ± 6	45 ± 10

[a] Monolayer cultures of 6-day C57BL/6J mouse cerebella were maintained *in vitro* for 2 days and then stained by double immunofluorescence for cell-type-specific markers as described in the text. For labeling of O antigens, live cells were used to assure staining of cell surfaces only.

mann glial processes were visible with O2 and O3 antibodies. Since in fresh-frozen sections of tissues the intracellular antigens as well as cell surface components are accessible to antibody, it seemed important to probe directly for the localization of the corresponding antigenic species under conditions where only cell surface constituents are identified. When antibodies are applied to live monolayer cultures of early postnatal mouse cerebellum so as to react with cell surface constituents only, none of the O antibodies reacts with the surfaces of astrocytes, neurons, fibroblasts, or fibroblastlike cells as determined by double immunodouble-labeling methods with cell-type-specific markers. Antigens O1 and O2 are expressed on galactocerebroside-positive cells (Table VI), whereas O3 and O4 antigens are present on additional cells which are negative for any of the markers tested. Electron-microscopic examination of immunoperoxidase-labeled cultures clearly shows that these cells are indeed oligodendroglia. When antibodies are applied to paraformaldehyde and ethanol- or acetone-fixed cultures, where intracellular antigens are accessible, O1, O2, and O3 antibodies label astrocytes in a GFA-protein-like pattern.

Table VII. *O Antigen Expression in Cultures of Embryonic Day 13 Pons and Cerebellum*

Days	01	02	03	04
1	−[a]	−	−	−
2	−	−	−	−
3	−	−	+[b]	+
4	±	+	+	+
5	+	+	+	+

[a] — refers to the absence of immunofluorescent cells.
[b] + refers to the detectability of immunofluorescent cells.

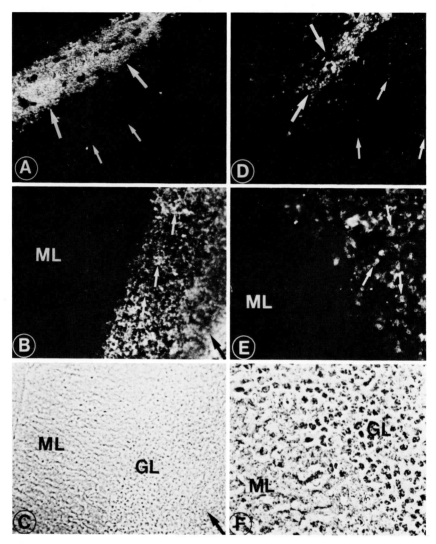

Figure 9. Immunolabeling for O antigens in fresh-frozen sagittal sections of adult C57BL/ 6J mouse cerebellum. (A, D) Antigen O1 is stained in white-matter tracts (large arrows). Some labeling is also seen in the granular layer (small arrows) at the end of a cerebellar folium. (B, E) Antigen O4 is stained in white matter (large arrow) and small vesicular structures in the granular layer (GL) (small arrows). Molecular layer (ML) is not stained. (C) and (F) are phase contrast micrographs to (B) and (E), respectively. (A, D, E, F) × 560; (B, C) × 220, reproduced at 75%. (From Sommer and Schachner, 1981b.)

O3 and O4 antigens are present on oligodendroglia which are less mature than galactocerebroside or NS1-antigen-bearing cells. On freshly trypsinized, viable single-cell suspensions of neonatal cerebellum, O3 and O4 antigens, but not O1 and O2 antigens, are detectable. At postnatal day 7 all O antigens are detectable. In monolayer cultures of fetal pons and cerebellum O3 and O4 antigens become detectable 1 day before O1 and O2 antigens (Table VII). In these cultures O3 and O4 antigens have the tendency to be expressed by more simple or immature looking cells, while O1- and O2-antigen-positive cells are found on more elaborate and slender process-bearing cells (Figs. 10 and 11). It is difficult, however, to judge from these morphological criteria alone whether a cell would belong to the group of more immature or mature oligodendroglia. After prolonged periods in culture more O3- and O4-antigen-positive cells express galactocerebroside than after shorter times in culture.

Evidence will be given that cells that are O1-antigen- or galactocerebroside-negative but O4-antigen-positive are direct precursors to O1 antigen or galactocerebroside-positive cells. O1-antigen-positive cells can be removed from single-cell suspensions by complement-dependent immunocytolysis. Residual O4-antigen-positive cells can then be isolated using magnetic beads coupled to O4 antibody (Meier *et al.*, 1981; Meier and Schachner, 1981). The isolated O4-antigen-positive, but O1-antigen-negative, cells are freed from the beads and maintained in culture for various time periods to monitor for O1 expression by indirect immunofluorescence. After 1 day of culture O1 antigen becomes detectable. In another type of experiment, O4-antigen-positive, but O1 antigen-negative cells obtained by immunocytolysis as described above are labeled with rhodamine-coupled O4 antibodies at the time of plating in culture. During the first hours *in vitro* the rhodamine label is internalized and newly appearing O1 antigen can be visualized by fluorescein-conjugated O1 antibody. Cells labeled by both fluorochromes can be seen after 6 hr (Sommer and Schachner, 1981*a*).

These observations establish the existence of cell surface markers for oligodendroglia at more immature developmental stages than have been recognized by previously established markers. These include NS-1 antigen, galactocerebroside, and myelin basic protein (Schachner and Willinger, 1979*a*). It is hoped that immunizations with this more immature oligodendroglial population will produce monoclonal antibodies that recognize even less mature oligodendroglial antigens which might still be expressed by the cell population used as antigen. By tracing antigenic markers back to even earlier stages it is conceivable that a genealogical tree will emerge that is composed of neuronal, astroglial

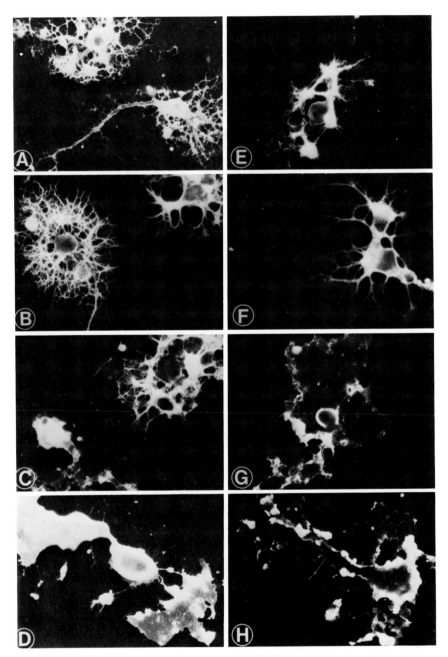

Figure 10. Immunolabeling of O antigens in cerebellar cultures of 7-day C57BL/6J mice. (A, G) Antigen O1; (B, C) antigen O4; (D, E, H) antigen O2; (F, G) antigen O3. × 560, reproduced at 65%. (From Schachner *et al.*, 1981.)

and oligodendroglial branches. The special shape of this tree should help determine the ontogenetic evolution of the individual glial cell types in the cerebellum.

It is difficult at present to estimate the significance of O-antigen expression on the cell surface of oligodendrocytes as well as in cytoplasma of astrocytes. It may suffice to say here that such cross-reactivities have also been observed using conventional polyclonal antibodies to sulfatide (Zalc et al., 1981) and monoclonal antibodies to oligodendrocyte cell surfaces (L. F. Reichardt, personal communication).

3. NEURONAL MARKERS

The recognition of immunological cell surface markers specific for individual neuronal subclasses is of prime importance for studying interactions between synaptogenesis and the five neuronal cerebellar cell types. In addition, cell surface markers specific for a particular developmental stage or for functional specializations at topographically distinct sizes within a particular cell type are called for. It would be desirable, for instance, to distinguish a granule cell which has just become postmitotic from one that extends axonal processes and is beginning its inward migration. Would it be possible to recognize a cell surface makeup on the leading process of a granule cell which is different from the surface composition of the axonal processes? Would it be possible to immunologically define a surface molecule on the leading process or cell body which interacts with a complementary molecular species on the Bergmann glial process just at the time of migration? If such cell surface constituents exist and can be recognized by immunological reagents, it would be feasible to determine whether such surface constituents are distributed uniformly over cell body and leading process or as a gradient. Unfortunately, our immunological methods have yet to give evidence of such a sophisticated level of discrimination.

At present, it is possible to distinguish neurons from other cell types by two cell surface constituents, NS4 antigen and tetanus toxin receptors, as has been mentioned earlier. Both of these markers have been found to be expressed in the neuroectoderm as early as embryonic day 11 in the mouse (Schnitzer and Schachner, 1979, 1981c; see also Berwald-Netter et al., 1980). At this age, they are present on cell types which are negative for any of the glial or fibroblastic markers. Direct proof, however, that only neurons or a special type of neuron is recognized at these early stages will have to come from combined electrophysiological, morphological, and immunological studies. At early postnatal ages, NS-4 antigen and tetanus toxin receptors seem to be present on all types of

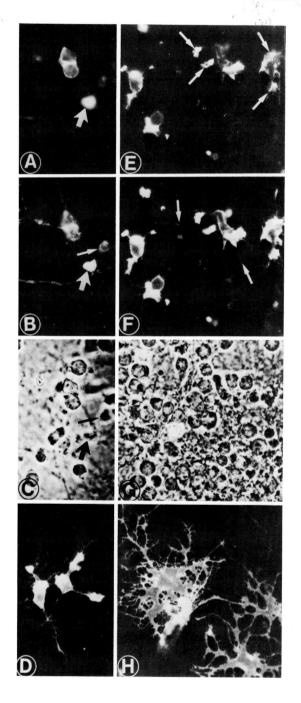

cerebellar neurons, and can be specifically detected *in vitro* under the appropriate culture conditions and *in vivo* in histological preparations by indirect immunofluorescence or immunoperoxidase methods (Schnitzer and Schachner, 1979, 1981a). This apparent cell type specificity is dependent on the sensitivity of the detection method. It is likely that glial cells or fibroblasts also contain the receptors for tetanus toxin, the higher gangliosides G_{D1b} and G_{T1} (Van Heyningen, 1963); they may be present on the cell surface of these cells at such low levels, however, that they remain undetectable by indirect immunocytological techniques. The characterization of a monoclonal antibody obtained from an immunization with bovine retina (J. Schnitzer *et al.*, unpublished results) has revealed another cell surface marker for neurons. In contrast to NS-4 antigen and tetanus toxin receptors, this antigen is present on neurons of the CNS, but not on neurons of the peripheral nervous system. It remains to be determined, however, whether all neuronal cerebellar cell types are recognized and at which developmental stages.

Although cholera toxin does not display a restricted preference for neurons, but also reacts with some, though not all astrocytes and oligodendrocytes in culture (Willinger and Schachner, 1978; Schachner and Willinger, 1979b; Raff *et al.*, 1979b), it has been a useful marker for distinguishing the degree of maturity of cerebellar neurons with a small cell body, most of which are granule cell neurons (see Table 1). It is possible that stellate and basket cells may also show this maturational difference. A demonstration of these neurons has, however, remained elusive to this point, since independent markers in the form of antiserum to GAD or neuron-specific GABA uptake have yet to be tested. The G_{M1} binding subunit of cholera toxin, choleragenoid, has been used in our experiments to rule out any interaction with adenylate cyclase. Toxin binding sizes are detected by exposure of target cells or tissue to toxin, followed by antitoxin antibody and finally by fluorescent antiimmunoglobulin label.

←———————————————————————————————

Figure 11. Immunolabeling of O3 antigen in cultures of pons and cerebellum from 13-day embryonic NMRI mice. O3 antigen was tested by indirect immunofluorescence after various days of culture. (A, B, C) Three days *in vitro*. Micrograph (A) shows labeled cell bodies in focus; cellular processes of these cells are focused upon in (B). Phase contrast micrograph to (A) and (B) is shown in (C) with focus on cell bodies. Of these, only two out of at least six are immunolabeled. Small, round structure in (B) and (C) (small arrows) is probably not a cell, but possibly a nucleus or membrane vesicle. Diffusely labeled debris is also seen (A, B, C) (large arrows). (E, F, G) four days *in vitro*. Micrograph (E) focuses on bristlelike structures emanating from cell body and processes (arrows). (F) is more in focus of cell bodies and more extended cellular processes (arrows). Phase contrast micrograph of (E) and (F) is shown in (G). (D) and (H) are 5 and 6 days *in vitro*, respectively. × 560, reproduced at 65%. (From Schachner *et al.*, 1981.)

Two lines of evidence support the notion that G_{M1} increases during development on granule cell neurons (Willinger and Schachner, 1980). Examination of histological sections reveals that the external side of the external granular layer of 8-day cerebellum is relatively unstained compared with the internal side consisting of postmitotic cells ready to migrate to the internal granular layer. In culture, another type of experiment was performed to correlate DNA synthesis, which takes place in the matrix zone of the external side of the external granular layer, and expression of G_{M1} ganglioside. Two groups of mice are injected with [³H]thymidine and sacrificed at postnatal day 8, which is either 3 hr or 3 days later. In the former case only the external matrix cells are autoradiographically labeled; in the latter, some cells in the inner part of the external granular layer, but mostly in the internal granular layer, are labeled. Cerebellar cells are cultured from mice labeled in this manner, and after 48 hr maintenance *in vitro* they are scored at the same time for autoradiographic grains and G_{M1} ganglioside by immunofluorescence. Cholera toxin cannot be detected on actively dividing cells (from mice after 3 hr of pulse labeling). However, 70% of the toxin-positive cells which have become postmitotic in the pulse-chase experiment (from mice 3 days after the thymidine pulse) contain thymidine. It seems, therefore, that observations both *in vivo* and *in vitro* support the concept that differentiation of granule cells (and possibly other neurons with small cell bodies) is accompanied by an increase in expression of G_{M1} ganglioside. It remains to be determined if G_{M1} expression is augmented uniformly over cell soma and processes, or if topographically distinct domains are differentially marked in the developing neuron.

Knowledge of the developmental sequence in appearance of a cell surface marker can also lead to a distinction of particular neuronal cell types. If a cell surface antigen appears only after a certain period has passed beyond its birthdate, a separation becomes possible on the basis of cell age. Thy-1 antigen (for references, see Schnitzer and Schachner, 1981a) is a candidate for this phenomenon. It can be shown that cerebellar neurons with large cell bodies, which are born between embryonic day 11 and 13, express Thy-1 antigen at early postnatal ages. Neurons with small cell bodies, which withdraw from the cell cycle only during the 1st and 2nd postnatal weeks, lack Thy-1 on their surface (Schnitzer and Schachner, 1981c). Large neurons labeled with [³H]thymidine at day 12 of gestation and separated at postnatal day 3 by BSA density gradient centrifugation to enrich for large and small neurons can be shown to carry autoradiographic grains also labeled for Thy-1 antigen (Schnitzer and Schachner, 1981b). Small neurons are devoid both of thymidine and Thy-1. A large proportion of these large neurons are Purkinje cells, but some of these are possibly also Golgi type II neurons.

Other cell types, such as fibroblasts or astroglia, which start to express Thy-1 antigen after several days of culture (Schnitzer and Schachner, 1981a), do not complicate the separation scheme, since at postnatal day 3, freshly dissociated large neurons are the only cells to express Thy-1 antigen.

4. CONCLUDING REMARKS

The characterization of intracellular and cell surface antigens in the mouse cerebellum has led to the recognition of several cell-type-specific markers and the delineation of their developmental expression. Although it has been possible to detect antigenic differences between the major subclasses of neural cell types, and between subsets of astro- and oligodendroglial cell populations, distinction between cerebellar neurons has so far been achieved solely on the basis of differences in differentiative stage among developing neurons.

Markers that distinguish among cerebellar neurons after completion of their differentiative program have remained elusive. It is hoped, however, that with the advent of monoclonal antibodies the refinement in deciphering the molecular individualities of cerebellar neurons will be pushed to further limits. It is also hoped that such unique cellular traits do indeed exist so they can be exploited for immunoselection of individual neuronal populations.

ACKNOWLEDGMENTS

The author wishes to express her gratitude to her colleagues and students who have participated in this work. Support from Land Baden-Württemberg, Deutsche Forschungsgemeinschaft, Stiftung Volkswagenwerk, and Gemeinnützige Hertie Stiftung is gratefully acknowledged.

5. REFERENCES

Altman, J., and Anderson, W. J., 1972, Experimental reorganization of the cerebellar cortex. I. Morphological effects of elimination of all microneurons with prolonged x-irradiation started at birth, J. Comp. Neurol. 146:355.

Berg, G., and Schachner, M., 1981, Immunoelectronmicroscopic identification of O antigen bearing oligodendroglial cells in vitro, Cell Tissue Res. 219:313.

Berwald-Netter, Y., Bizzini, B., Couraud, F., Koulakoff, A., Martin-Montot, N., 1980, Specific surface membrane markers as probes for neuronal evolution in vivo and in vitro. I. Meeting of the International Society for Devel. Neuroscience, p. 279.

Bignami, A., Eng. L. F., Dahl, D., and Uyeda, C. T., 1972, Localization of the glial fibrillary acidic protein in astrocytes by immunofluorescence, *Brain Res.* **43**:429.

Campbell, G. LeM., Schachner, M., and Sharrow, S. O., 1977, Isolation of glial cell-enriched and -depleted populations from mouse cerebellum by density gradient centrifugation and electronic cell sorting, *Brain Res.* **127**:69.

Caviness, V., and Rakic, P., 1978, Mechanisms of cortical development: A view from mutations in mice, *Ann. Rev. Neurosci.* **1**:297.

Das, G. D., 1974, Contact guidance and migratory cells in the developing cerebellum, *Brain Res.* **69**:13.

Dimpfel, W., Huang, R. T. C., and Habermann, I., 1977, Gangliosides in nervous tissue and binding of ^{125}I-labelled tetanus toxin, a neuronal marker, *J. Neurochem.* **29**:329.

Eccles, J., Ito, M., and Szentágothai, J., 1967, *The Cerebellum as a Neuronal Machine*, Springer, Berlin.

Egar, M., and Singer, M., 1972, The role of ependyma in spinal cord regeneration in the urodele, Triturus, *J. Exp. Neurol.* **37**:422.

Eng, L. F., Vanderhaegen, J. J., Bignami, B., and Gerstl, B., 1971, An acidic protein isolated from fibrous astrocytes, *Brain Res.* **28**:351.

Falconer, D. S., 1951, Two new mutants "trembler" and "reeler" with neurological actions in the house mouse (*Mus musculus*), *J. Genet.* **50**:192.

Franke, W. W., Schmid, E., Osborn, M., Weber, K., 1978, Different intermediate-sized filaments distinguished by immunofluorescence microscopy, *Proc. Natl. Acad. Sci. U.S.A.* **75**:5034.

Franke, W. W., Schmid, E., Osborn, M., and Weber, K., 1979, Intermediate-sized filaments of human endothelial cells, *J. Cell Biol.* **81**:570.

Fujita, S., 1967, Quantitative analysis of cell proliferation and differentiation in the cortex of the postnatal mouse cerebellum, *J. Cell Biol.* **32**:277.

Fujita, S., Shimada, M., and Nakamura, I., 1966, ^{3}H-Thymidine autoradiographic studies on the cell proliferation and differentiation in the external and internal granular layers of the mouse cerebellum, *J. Comp. Neurol.* **128**:191.

Herndon, R. M., 1968, Thiophen induced granule cell necrosis in the rat cerebellum, *Exp. Brain Res.* **6**:49.

Herndon, R. M., Margolis, G., and Kilham, L,, 1971a, The synaptic organization of the malformed cerebellum induced by perinatal infection with the feline panleukopenia virus (PLV). I. Elements forming the cerebellar glomeruli, *J. Neuropathol. Exp. Neurol.* **30**:196.

Herndon, R. M., Margolis, G., and Kilham, L., 1971b, The synaptic organization of the malformed cerebellum induced by perinatal infection with the feline panleukopenia virus (PLV), II. The Purkinje cell and its afferents, *J. Neuropathol. Exp. Neurol.* **30**:557.

Hicks, S. P., 1954, The effects of ionizing radiation, certain hormones, and radiomimetric drugs on the developing nervous system, *J. Cell. Comp. Physiol.* **43**(Suppl. 1):151.

Hicks, S. P., and D'Amato, C. J., 1966, Effects of ionizing radiations on mammalian development, in: *Advances in Teratology* (D. H. M. Woollam, ed.), pp. 196–250, Logos, London.

Hirano, A., Dembitzer, H. M., 1973, Cerebellar alteration in the weaver mouse, *J. Cell Biol.* **56**:478.

His, W., 1889, Neuroblasten und deren Entstehung im embryonalen Mark, *Abhandl. Kgl. Saechs. Ges. Wiss. Math. Phys. Kl.* **15**:313.

Huntington, H. W., and Terry, R. D., 1966, The origin of the reactive cells in cerebral stab wounds, *J. Neuropathol. Exp. Neurol.* **25**:646.

Kilham, L., and Margolis, G., 1966a, Viral etiology of spontaneous ataxia of cats, *Am. J. Pathol.* **48**:991.

Kilham, L., and Margolis, G., 1966b, Spontaneous hepatitis and cerebellar "hypoplasia" in suckling rats due to congenital infections with rat virus, *Am. J. Pathol.* **49**:457.

Köhler, G., and Milstein, C., 1975, Continuous cultures of fused cells secreting antibody of predefined specificity, *Nature (London)* **256**:495.

Köhler, G., and Milstein, C., 1976, Derivation of specific antibody-producing tissue culture and tumor lines by cell fusion, *Eur. J. Immunol.* **6**:511.

Korte, G. E., and Rosenbluth, J., 1980, Membrane specializations in frog ependymal astrocytes, 10th Annual Meeting, Society for Neuroscience, *Abstract* **247**:16.

Kuffler, S., and Nicholls, J. G., 1976, *From Neuron to Brain*, Sinauer Associates, Sunderland, Mass.

Lagenaur, C., Sommer, I., and Schachner, M., 1980, Subclass of astroglia recognized in mouse cerebellum by monoclonal antibody, *Dev. Biol.* **79**:367.

Lagenaur, C., Master, C., and Schachner, M., 1981, Changes in expression of glial antigens M1 and C1 after cerebellar injury, *J. Neuroscience*, in press.

Landis, S. C., Mullen, R. J., 1978, The development and degeneration of Purkinje cells in pcd mutant mice, *J. Comp. Neurol.* **177**:125.

Landis, D. M. D., Reese, T. S., 1977, Structure of the Purkinje cell membrane in staggerer and weaver mutant mouse. *J. Comp. Neurol.* **171**:247.

Landis, D. M. D., Sidman, R. L., 1974, Cerebellar cortical development in the staggerer mouse, *J. Neuropathol. Exp. Neurol.* **33**:180.

Lane, P., 1964, Personal communication in *Mouse News Letter* **30**:32.

Llinás, R., 1969, Neurobiology of cerebellar evolution and development, *Proceedings of the First International Symposium of the Institute for Biomedical Research*, AMA Educational Research Foundation, Chicago, IL.

Mareš, V., Lodin, Z., and Srajer, J., 1970, The cellular kinetics of the developing mouse cerebellum. I. The generation cycle, growth fraction and rate of proliferation of the external granular layer, *Brain Res.* **23**:323.

Mariani, J., Crepel, F., Mikoshiba, K., Changeux, J.-P., Sotelo, C., 1977, Anatomical, physiological and biochemical studies of the cerebellum from reeler mutant mouse, *Philos. Trans. R. Soc. London* **281**:1.

Maxwell, D. S., and Krüger, L., 1965, The fine structure of astrocytes in the cerebral cortex and their response to focal injury produced by heavy ionizing particles, *J. Cell Biol.* **25**:141.

Meier, D. H., and Schachner, M., 1982, Immunoselection of oligodendrocytes by magnetic beads. II. *In vitro* maintenance of immunoselected oligodendrocytes, *J. Neuroscience Res.*, in press.

Meier, D. H., Lagenaur, C., and Schachner, M., 1982, Immunoselection of oligodendrocytes by magnetic beads. I. Determination of antibody coupling parameters and cell binding conditions, *J. Neuroscience Res.*, in press.

Miale, I. L., and Sidman, R. L., 1961, An autoradiographic analysis of histogenesis in the mouse cerebellum, *Exp. Neurol.* **4**:277.

Mirsky, R., Wendon, L., Black, P., Stolkin, C., and Bray, D., 1978, Tetanus toxin: A cell surface marker for neurones in culture, *Brain Res.* **148**:251.

Mugnaini, E., and Forströnen, P. F., 1967, Ultrastructural studies on the cerebellar histogenesis. I. Differentiation of granule cells and development of glomeruli in the chick embryo, *Z. Zellforsch. Mikrosk. Anat. Abt. Histochem.* **77**:115.

Mullen, R. J., and LaVail, M. M., 1975, Two new types of retinal degeneration in cerebellar mutant mice, *Nature (London)* **258**:528.

Mullen, R. J., Eicher, E. M., and Sidman, R. L., 1976, Purkinje cell degeneration, a new neurological mutation in the mouse, *Proc. Natl. Acad. Sci. U.S.A.* **73**:208.

Nathanson, N., Cole, G. A., and Van der Loos, H., 1969, Heterotopic cerebellar granule cells following administration of cyclophosphamide to suckling rats, *Brain Res.* **15**:532.

Nieuwenhuys, R., 1964, Comparative anatomy of the cerebellum, *Progr. Brain Res.* **25**:1.

Nordlander, R. H., and Singer, M., 1978, The role of ependyma in regenaration of the spinal cord in the urodele amphibian tail, *J. Comp. Neurol.* **180(2)**:349.

Oksche, A., 1980, *Neuroglia I*, Springer-Verlag, Berlin.

Palay, S., and Chan-Palay, V., 1974, *Cerebellar Cortex Cytology and Organization*, Springer-Verlag, New York.

Peters, A., Palay, S. L., and DeF. Webster, H., 1976, *The Fine Structure of the Nervous System*. The Neurons and Supporting *Cells, Saunders*, Philadelphia.

Privat, A., 1975, Postnatal gliogenesis in the mammalian brain, *Int. Rev. Cytol.* **40**:281.

Raaf, J., and Kernohan, J. W., 1944, A study of the external granular layer in the cerebellum, *Am. J. Anat.* **75**:151.

Raff, M. C., Brockes, J. P., Fields, K. L., and Mirsky, R., 1979a, Neural cell markers, the end of the beginning, *Progr. Brain Res.* **51**:17.

Raff, M. C., Fields, K. L., Hakomori, S., Mirsky, R., Pruss, R. M., and Winter, J., 1979b, Cell type-specific markers for distinguishing and studying neurons and the major classes of glial cells in culture, *Brain Res.* **174**:283.

Rakic, P., 1971, Neuron-glia relationship during granule cell migration in developing cerebellar cortex: A Golgi and electronmicroscopic study in *Macacus thesus, J. Comp. Neurol.* **141**:283.

Rakic, P., 1972, Extrinsic cytological determinants of basket and stellate cell dendritic pattern in the cerebellar molecular layer, *J. Comp. Neurol.* **146**:335.

Rakic, P., 1973, Kinetics of proliferation and latency between final cell division and onset of differentiation of cerebellar stellate and basket neurons, *J. Comp. Neurol.* **147**:523.

Rakic, P., and Sidman, R. L., 1973, Organization of cerebellar cortex secondary to deficit of granule cells in weaver mutant mice, *J. Comp. Neurol.* **152**:133.

Ramón y Cajal, S., 1909–1911, *Histologie du Système Nerveux de l'Homme et des Vertébrés*, 2 vols. (L. Azoulay, trans.). (Reprinted by Instituto Ramón y Cajal del C.S.I.C., Madrid, 1952–1955).

Ramón y Cajal, S., 1955, *Histologie du Système Nerveux*, vol 2, C.S.I.C., Madrid.

Rezai, Z., Yoon, C. H., 1972, Abnormal rate of granule cell migration in the cerebellum of "weaver" mutant mice, *Dev. Biol.* **29**:17.

Rohrer, H., and Schachner, M., 1980, Surface proteins of cultured mouse cerebellar cells, *J. Neurochem.* **35**:792.

Schachner, M., and Willinger, M., 1979a, Developmental expression of oligodendrocyte specific cell surface markers: NS-1 (nervous system antigen-1), cerebroside, and basic protein of myelin, in: *The Menarini Series on Immunopathology* P. A. Miescher, L. Bolis, S. Gorini, T. A. Lambo, G. J. V. Nossal, and G. Torrigiani, eds.), vol. 2, pp. 37–60.

Schachner, M., and Willinger, M., 1979b, Cell type specific cell surface antigens in the cerebellum, *Prog. Brain Res.* **51**:23.

Schachner, M., Wortham, K. A., Carter, L. D., and Chaffee, J. K., 1975, NS-4 (nervous system antigen-4), a cell surface antigen of developing and adult mouse brain and mature sperm, *Dev. Biol.* **44**:313.

Schachner, M., Wortham, K. A., Ruberg, M. Z., Dorfman, S., and LeM. Campbell, G., 1977, Brain cell surface antigens detected by anti-corpus callosum antiserum, *Brain Res.* **127**:87.

Schachner, M., Smith, C., and Schoonmaker, G., 1978a, Immunological distinction between neurofilament and glial fibrillary acidic proteins by mouse antisera and their immunohistological distribution, *Dev. Neurosci.* **1:**1.

Schachner, M., Schoonmaker, G., and Hynes, R. O., 1978*b*, Cellular and subscellular localization of LETS protein in the nervous system, *Brain Res.* **158:**149.

Schachner, M., Kim, S. K., and Zehnle, R., 1981, Developmental expression in central and peripheral nervous system of oligodendrocyte cell surface antigens (O antigens) recognized by monoclonal antibodies, *Dev. Biol.* **83:**328.

Schaper, A., 1897*a*, Die frühesten Differenzierungsvorgänge im Centralnervensystem, *Arch. Entwicklungsmech. Org.* **5:**81.

Schaper, A., 1897*b*, The earliest differentiation in the central nervous system of vertebrates, *Science* **5:**430.

Schmechel, D. E., and Rakic, P., 1979, A Golgi study of radial glial cells in developing monkey telencephalon: Morphogenesis and transformation into astrocytes, *Anat. Embryol.* **156:**115.

Schnitzer, J., and Schachner, M., 1979, Isolation and characterization of cell populations of early postnatal mouse cerebellar cortex *in vitro*, VII International Meeting of the International Society of Neurochemistry, Jerusalem.

Schnitzer, J., and Schachner, M., 1981*a*, Expression of Thy-1, H-2 and NS-4 cell surface antigens and tetanus toxin receptors in early postnatal and adult mouse cerebellum, *J. Neuroimmunol.* **1:**429.

Schnitzer, J., and Schachner, M., 1981*b*, Characterization of isolated mouse cerebellar cell populations *in vitro*, *J. Neuroimmunol.* **1:**457.

Schnitzer, J., and Schachner, M., 1981*c*, Developmental expression of cell type-specific markers in mouse cerebellar cortical cells *in vitro*, *J. Neuroimmunol.* **1:**471.

Schnitzer, J., Franke, W. W., and Schachner, M., 1981, Immunocytochemical demonstration of vimentin in astrocytes and ependymal cells of developing and adult mouse nervous system, *J. Cell Biol.* **90:**435.

Shimada, M., and Langman, J., 1970, Repair of the external granular layer after postnatal treatment with 5-fluorodeoxyuridine, *Am. J. Anat.* **129:**247.

Sidman, R. L., 1968, Development of interneuronal connections in brains of mutant mice, in: *Physiological and Biochemical Aspects of Nervous Integration* (F. D. Carlson, ed.), pp. 163–193, Prentice-Hall, Englewood Cliffs, N.J.

Sidman, R. L., Lane, P. W., Dickie, M. M., 1962, Staggerer, a new mutation in the mouse cerebellum, *Science* **137:**610.

Sidman, R. L., Green, M. C., and Appel, S. H., 1965, *Catalog of the Neurological Mutants of the Mouse*, p. 82, Harvard University Press, Cambridge, Mass.

Smart, I., and Leblond, C. P., 1961, Evidence for division and transformation of neuroglia cells in the mouse brain as derived from radioautography after injection of ^{3}H-thymidine, *J. Comp. Neurol.* **116:**349.

Sommer, I., and Schachner, M., 1981*a*, O4 antigen-positive and O1 antigen-negative cells are precursors of O1 antigen-positive oligodendrocytes, submitted for publication.

Sommer, I., and Schachner, M., 1981*b*, Monoclonal antibodies (O1 to O4) to oligodendrocyte cell surfaces: An immunocytological study in the central nervous system, *Dev. Biol.* **83:**311.

Sommer, I., and Schachner, M., 1981*c*, Expression of glial antigens C1 and M1 in developing and adult neurologically mutant mice, *J. Supramol. Struct.*, in press.

Sommer, I., Lagenaur, C., and Schachner, M., 1981, Recognition of Bergmann glial and ependymal cells in the mouse nervous system by monoclonal antibody, *J. Cell Biol.* **90:**448.

Sotelo, C., 1975*a*, Dendritic abnormalities of Purkinje cells in cerebellum of neurological mutant mice (weaver and staggerer), *Adv. Neurol.* **12:**335.

Sotelo, C., 1975b, Anatomical, physiological and biochemical studies of cerebellum from mutant mice. II. Morphological study of cerebellar cortical neurons and circuits in the weaver mouse, Brain Res. 94:19.

Sotelo, C., Changeux, J.-P., 1974a, Transsynaptic degeneration "en cascade" in the cerebellar cortex of staggerer mutant mice, Brain Res. 67:519.

Sotelo, C., Changeux, J.-P., 1974b, Bergmann fibers and granular cell migration in the cerebellum of homozygous weaver mutant mouse, Brain Res. 77:484.

Tapscott, S. J., Bennett, G. S., and Holtzer, H., 1980, Transition between intermediate filament types during neurogenesis, J. Cell Biol. 87:181a.

Timpl, R., Rohde, H., Robey, P. G., Rennard, S. I., Foidart, J.-M., and Martin, G. R., 1979, Laminin—A glycoprotein from basement membranes, J. Biol. Chem. 254:9933.

Uzman, L. L., 1960, The histogenesis of the mouse cerebellum as studied by its tritiated thymidine uptake, J. Comp. Neurol. 114:137.

Van Heyningen, W. E., 1963, The fixation of tetanus toxin, strychnine, serotonin and other substances by ganglioside, J. Gen. Microbiol. 31:375.

Vaughn, J. E., Hinds, P. L., and Skoff, R. P., 1970. Electron microscopic studies of Wallerian degeneration in rat optic nerves. I. The mutipotential glia, J. Comp. Neurol. 140:175.

Webster, W., Shimada, M., and Langman, J., 1973, Effect of fluorodeoxyuridine, colcemid, and bromodeoxyuridine on developing neocortex of the mouse, Am. J. Anat. 137:67.

Willinger, M., and Schachner, M., 1978, Distribution of G_{M1} ganglioside in developing cerebellum, J. Supramol. Struct. Suppl. 2:128.

Willinger, M., and Schachner, M., 1980, G_{M1} ganglioside as a marker for neuronal differentiation in mouse cerebellum, Devel. Biol. 74:101.

Zalc, B., Monge, M., Dupouey, P., Hauw, J. J., and Baumann, N. A., 1981, Immunohistochemical localization of galactosyl- and sulfogalactosylceramide in the brain of 30-day-old mouse, Brain Res. 211:341.

Zamenhof, S., Grauel, L., and van Marthens, E., 1971, The effect of thymidine and 5-bromodeoxyuridine on developing chick embryo brain, Res. Commun. Chem. Pathol. Pharmacol. 2:261.

Index